COOKING WITH
◆ YOGURT ◆

COOKING WITH
◆ YOGURT ◆

The Complete Cookbook for Indulging

with the World's Healthiest Food

JUDITH CHOATE

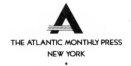

THE ATLANTIC MONTHLY PRESS
NEW YORK
◆

Published simultaneously in Canada
Printed in the United States of America
FIRST EDITION

Library of Congress Cataloging-in-Publication Data

Choate, Judith.
Cooking with yogurt: the complete cookbook for indulging with the world's healthiest food / Judith Choate.—1st ed.
Includes index.
ISBN 0-87113-566-3
1. Cookery (Yogurt)   I. Title.
TX759.5.Y63C49   1994   641.6′7146—dc20   93-33785

DESIGN BY LAURA HOUGH

The Atlantic Monthly Press
841 Broadway
New York, NY 10003

2 4 6 8 10 9 7 5 3 1

◆ CONTENTS ◆

COOKING WITH
◆ YOGURT ◆

◆ INTRODUCTION ◆

I love yogurt—its taste, texture, and versatility enthrall me. I started cooking with it simply because I always had it on hand. Well into preparing breakfast or dinner, making breads or desserts, or readying for a party, I would often find myself out of eggs or milk or oil. Yogurt became the cure-all to avoid culinary disasters. The fact that it was usually nonfat and unflavored made it an even better addition to my kitchen and to my continual quest for recipes that would provide low- or nonfat dishes and reduced cholesterol meals.

Beginning with biblical references up through the international cuisine of the nineties, yogurt has been "the" constant kitchen cure-all. One of nature's original prepared foods, yogurt was probably discovered by the nomadic tribes of the Far East when the milk carried in their sheepskin pouches inadvertently fermented from the sun's warmth. This could, however, just be another tale in the rather fanciful history of yogurt, which begins with Abraham being taught to make yogurt by an angel! Even with all of the twentieth century's scientific advances, the magic of yogurt is still believed to be the root of the extraordinary longevity of the people of the Caucasus and Bulgaria.

Is yogurt truly the ideal food? Undoubtedly not! If you eat yogurt made from rich milk with a high fat content you will be eating yogurt just as rich and just as high in fat. However, if you eat nonfat yogurt, you will get just that—no fat and no cholesterol as well as the fewest calories you will find in any substitute for heavy or sour cream, creamy cheese, mayonnaise, or salad dressing. I have taken its use a step further and often use it as a replacement for eggs and/or oil when cooking for my family. Ideal? No, but certainly better for you than its richer counterparts. It also has the benefit of being high in vitamins, protein, calcium, and riboflavin and is more easily digested by those who are lactose intolerant.

Except for its use in a few ethnic cuisines and by health food "nuts," yogurt was virtually unknown in the United States until the 1960s. Whether it was because of the influence of the back-to-nature Woodstock generation or the enthusiastic promotion of a "new" product by the dairy industry, yogurt became America's fastest-growing foodstuff. It now has a higher per capita consumption than milk: Yogurt, or laban, as it is frequently called throughout the rest of the world, is now more commonplace than Elsie the Cow!

Yogurt is made from pasteurized milk that has been injected with a specific bacteria. During the incubation process the bacteria thrive on lactose (milk sugar), producing lactic acid, which gives yogurt its distinct, slightly sour taste. The type of milk used and how long it is allowed to ferment will also determine the thickness and acidity of the final yogurt.

Yogurt can easily be made at home with or without a yogurt maker. The basic method I use is given on pages 6–7. However, there are also many superb yogurts available in both the supermarket dairy section and specialty food stores. Sheep's and goat's milk varieties have joined the now traditional cow's milk, with all of them offering a wide selection and some of them containing added sweeteners and/or natural flavors. The fat content will also vary greatly. To get the best nutritional value try to purchase unflavored yogurt made with the least amount of fat and with live, active cultures, free of preservatives, stabilizers, and artificial coloring agents.

In addition to its nutritional value, yogurt has many advocates for its use as a medicinal foodstuff. People on antibiotics are often told to eat yogurt to aid in the restoration of the beneficial intestinal bacteria destroyed by potent medication. For centuries, women have used yogurt to cure vaginal yeast infections and also as a beauty mask to rejuvenate facial skin. Intestinal disorders, ulcers, bowel and bladder infections, and many bacterial infections are often helped by a daily dietary regimen that includes a cup of yogurt. In fact, the therapeutic uses of yogurt are almost as varied as those in the kitchen.

COOKING WITH YOGURT

There are certain simple rules to follow when cooking with yogurt. Following them should ensure a nutritious and appetizing result.

1. The fresher the yogurt the better the result.

2. Never add cold yogurt to a hot mixture as it will separate into curds and whey. To prevent separation, before whisking into a hot (but not boiling) mixture, either bring yogurt to room temperature or mix yogurt with cornstarch (1/3 cup yogurt blended with 1 teaspoon cornstarch which has been dissolved in 1 tablespoon cold water).

3. Never boil a mixture to which yogurt has been added as the high heat will cause separation and kill the beneficial bacteria in the yogurt.

4. The more intense the heat, the less intense the healthy bacteria count. For example, baking kills all bacteria. Therefore, when possible, it is best to add the yogurt near the end of the cooking process.

5. Yogurt incorporates best when gently folded or whisked into mixtures.

6. If, after the addition of yogurt, your mixture is too thin, allow it to chill for at least an hour and it will, generally, thicken.

7. Whole milk, low-fat, and nonfat yogurt can be used interchangeably but the consistency and/or texture will vary, with whole milk being the thickest and most moist.

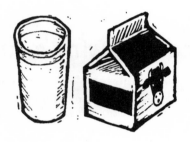

NUTRITIONAL CHART

The figures below have been taken from the labels of nationally distributed products. Specialty or gourmet varieties may vary in measure.

	Calories	Fat (g)	Calcium (mg)	Protein (g)	Cholesterol (mg)
Unflavored nonfat yogurt, 1 cup	110	0	430	11	Less than 5
Unflavored low-fat yogurt, 1 cup	140	4	430	10	15
Unflavored whole milk yogurt, 1 cup	140	7	274	10	29
Skim milk, 1 cup	80	1	290	8	10
Whole milk, 1 cup	150	8	390	10	35
Heavy cream, 1 cup	830	90	160	5	335
Sour cream, 1 cup	415	40	225	6	80
Cream cheese, 1 cup	790	79	185	17	250
Small curd creamed cottage cheese, 1 cup	215	9	125	26	30
Mayonnaise, 1 cup	1585	176	30	3	130
Butter, 1 cup	1730	195	50	2	530
Margarine, 1 cup	1630	182	70	2	0

MAKING YOGURT

Homemade yogurt is quick to prepare but slow to ferment. All you need is milk, enough heat to bring it to a boil, yogurt starter, and time.

It's best to use the freshest milk you can obtain. Fresh milk and yogurt products purchased directly from a local small dairy will generally be fresher than those from a supermarket. You should also use the same type of milk as yogurt starter—whole milk, whole milk yogurt starter; low-fat milk, low-fat yogurt starter; nonfat milk, nonfat yogurt starter.

The yogurt starter is simply a few spoonfuls of fresh yogurt. It may be purchased or homemade yogurt but, above all, it should be no more than two days old.

When making nonfat yogurt you may wish to add agar to the starter to help create a thicker, smoother, more flavorful yogurt. Agar is a gelling agent derived from marine algae which is easily obtained in either flaked, powdered, or granular form from health food stores.

◆ HOMEMADE YOGURT ◆

Makes 4 cups

4 cups milk (whole, low-, or nonfat)
2 tablespoons nonfat dry milk powder
3 tablespoons yogurt (whole, low-, or nonfat)
1 teaspoon agar, optional (available in health food stores)

Combine milk and milk powder in a medium saucepan over high heat. Stir to dissolve powder and bring to a boil. Immediately remove from heat and pour into a clean, nonporous container. Combine yogurt starter, agar, and about 1/2 cup of the boiled milk and stir to blend. Carefully stir yogurt mixture into the remaining milk. Cover with plastic wrap and place in a warm, draft-free spot (an oven with a pilot light is perfect) to rest undisturbed for 8 hours. Alternatively, place in an electric yogurt maker and follow manufacturer's instructions or in a preheated wide-mouth thermos.

When yogurt has set, remove it from the warm spot. Stir to blend. Cover and refrigerate until ready to use.

Note: *If the yogurt is too thin the incubation heat was probably too low. If the yogurt tastes too sour the incubation heat was probably too high. If either happens use the yogurt mixture for cooking or baking and try again!*

HOMEMADE YOGURT
◆ CHEESE ◆

Yogurt cheese isn't really cheese. It is simply yogurt that has been drained of most of its liquid to form a soft, spreadable yogurt not unlike cream cheese, for which it is a terrific replacement! One cup yogurt will yield approximately 1/3 cup yogurt cheese.

Line a sieve or colander with a piece of damp muslin, a triple layer of damp cheesecloth, or any other clean, moist, white cotton cloth, or use a pliable plastic funnel made especially for this purpose.

Pour yogurt into the prepared sieve or colander and place it over a bowl to drain for 8 hours for soft cheese, or up to 12 hours for very firm cheese.

When cheese has set, remove from cloth and gently press into desired shape or container. Cover and refrigerate. Yogurt cheese will keep, covered and refrigerated, for up to 1 week.

Do not discard drained yogurt liquid (the nutrient-rich whey), as it can be used as a replacement for milk or water in almost any recipe.

Variation: *Any flavored yogurt (such as lemon or vanilla) can be used to make cheese as long as it contains no gelatin or chopped fruit.*

◆ FROMAGE BLANC ◆

Makes 2 cups

This is a simple version of the French low-fat cheese often used as a thickener in low-calorie sauces. It can also be served with fruit or desserts in place of heavy cream.

1 cup fresh yogurt cheese
1 cup fresh yogurt
1 tablespoon fresh lemon juice

Place all ingredients in a food processor fitted with the metal blade. Using quick on/off turns, process until smooth. Cover and refrigerate. Fromage blanc will keep, covered and refrigerated, for up to 1 week.

IMITATION
◆ SOUR CREAM ◆

Makes 1 cup

1 cup 1% cottage cheese
1/4 cup low-fat plain yogurt
1/2 teaspoon fresh lemon juice or white vinegar

Combine all ingredients in a food processor fitted with the metal blade, or in a blender, and process until very smooth and thick. If mixture is too thick, thin with buttermilk, 1 teaspoon at a time.

HORS D'OEUVRES AND
◆ APPETIZERS ◆

Flavored Yogurt Cheese

Marinated Yogurt Cheese

Liptauer Cheese Canapés

Smoked Salmon Mousse in Tomato Cups

Herbed Spinach Balls with Mustard Dip

Deviled Eggs

Tzatziki

Cocktail Koftas

Baba Ghanooj

Easy and Low-fat Hummus

Crudités with 3 Dips
Roasted Red Pepper Dip
Curry Dip
Spicy Southwestern Dip

Indonesian Shrimp Barbecue with Mango Puree

FLAVORED YOGURT
◆ CHEESE ◆

Makes approximately 2 cups

2 cups Yogurt Cheese (page 8)
Coarse salt to taste

WITH FINE HERBS:
2 tablespoons each minced fresh parsley, chives, chervil,
   and tarragon

WITH LEMON PEPPER:
3 tablespoons freshly grated lemon zest
1 tablespoon freshly grated orange zest
1 tablespoon freshly ground black pepper or to taste

WITH GARLIC AND DILL:
3 cloves garlic, peeled and minced
2 tablespoons minced fresh dill

WITH SMOKED FISH:
1/2 cup chopped smoked salmon, trout, bluefish or any
   other moist smoked fish
1 small shallot, peeled and minced
1 teaspoon minced fresh parsley or dill, optional
Dash Tabasco

For each flavored cheese, gently mix all ingredients into cheese. Do not place in a food processor or beat vigorously. Shape blended cheese into a disk, place in a piece of plastic wrap, and close tightly. You may also pack it into a decorative serving dish and seal tightly. Or you may roll the shaped cheese on a mixture of minced herbs or parsley. Refrigerate for at least 8 hours to allow flavors to combine before serving.

Serve with crackers, toast points, pita or other chips, or any crisp flatbread, or with sliced fresh radishes and black bread. Flavored yogurt cheeses also make tasty tea sandwiches alone or with the addition of thinly sliced cucumbers.

MARINATED YOGURT
◆ CHEESE ◆

Makes approximately 2 cups

2 cups Yogurt Cheese (page 8)
3/4 cup extra virgin olive oil
2 tablespoons minced garlic
1 tablespoon minced shallot
2 tablespoons julienned fresh basil
1 tablespoon minced fresh rosemary
1 tablespoon minced fresh thyme
1 teaspoon minced fresh sage
1/2 teaspoon fresh lemon zest
Coarse salt to taste
Dried red pepper flakes to taste

Shape yogurt cheese into small disks and place them in a shallow, nonreactive dish. Combine remaining ingredients and pour over cheese. Cover and refrigerate for at least 12 hours before serving. Allow to come to room temperature and serve with crisp toast or any crisp cracker.

Note: *These disks are great warmed a bit under the broiler and served on top of a green salad.*

LIPTAUER CHEESE
◆ CANAPÉS ◆

Makes approximately 1 3/4 cups

1 cup Yogurt Cheese (page 8)
1/2 cup unsalted butter or margarine, softened
1/2 tablespoon minced anchovy filet or anchovy paste
1 1/2 tablespoons chopped fresh chives
1 teaspoon Worcestershire sauce
1 teaspoon minced capers
1 teaspoon dry mustard
1/2 teaspoon caraway seeds
1/2 teaspoon hot paprika
Dash Tabasco
36 toast rounds
1/4 cup minced fresh parsley

Combine all ingredients, except toast rounds and parsley, then mound cheese onto toast rounds. Sprinkle with parsley and serve immediately.

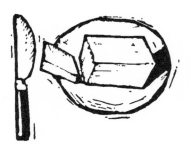

SMOKED SALMON MOUSSE
◆ IN TOMATO CUPS ◆

Makes 4 large or 24 small cups

3 cups Yogurt Cheese (page 8)
1/2 cup (4 ounces) cream cheese
3 ounces smoked salmon
2 tablespoons heavy cream
1 teaspoon fresh lemon juice
1/2 teaspoon fresh ginger juice (see Note below)
Dash Tabasco
4 medium tomatoes or approximately 24 cherry
    tomatoes
Minced fresh chives and dill or parsley sprigs for garnish

Place cheeses, salmon, cream, lemon and ginger juices, and Tabasco in a food processor fitted with the metal blade and process until smooth. Scrape into a pastry tube fitted with a large decorative tip. Refrigerate until ready to use. Wash tomatoes and cut off tops and completely clean out seeds and pulp. (A melon baller is a great device for speeding this process along.) Turn tomatoes upside down on a wire rack or a double layer of paper towels and allow to drain about 10 minutes.

When well-drained, turn over and pipe cheese mixture into each cavity. When all the tomatoes are filled, garnish tops with minced chives and a sprig of dill or parsley.

If serving as an appetizer, place on a bed of California spinach leaves.

Note: *For fresh ginger juice, grate fresh ginger root on the finest holes of a hand grater onto a double layer of cheesecloth. Tightly wrap the cloth around the grated ginger and extract the juice into a measuring spoon.*

HERBED SPINACH BALLS
◆ WITH MUSTARD DIP ◆

Makes approximately 36 balls

One 10-ounce package frozen chopped spinach, thawed
 and squeezed dry
1 cup herbed stuffing mix, finely crushed
1/2 cup grated Parmesan cheese
2 large egg whites
2 tablespoons melted unsalted butter or canola oil
2 tablespoons nonfat plain yogurt
2 tablespoons minced shallots
1 clove garlic, peeled and minced
1/2 teaspoon minced fresh sage
1/2 teaspoon minced fresh thyme
Salt and pepper to taste
Mustard Dip (recipe follows)

Preheat oven to 350°F.

Combine spinach, stuffing mix, cheese, egg whites, butter, yogurt, shallots, garlic, herbs, salt, and pepper, then shape into 1-inch balls. Set balls on a baking sheet, place in oven, and bake for about 10 minutes or until just golden. Remove from oven and drain on paper towels.

Serve warm with mustard dip.

◆ Mustard Dip ◆

Makes 1 1/4 cups

1 cup plain nonfat yogurt
1/4 cup honey mustard
Tabasco to taste

Combine all ingredients and refrigerate until ready to serve.

◆ DEVILED EGGS ◆

Makes 12 pieces

6 large hard-boiled eggs, peeled
3 tablespoons finely minced sun-dried tomatoes packed
   in oil
6 tablespoons plain nonfat yogurt
6 capers, finely minced
1 teaspoon minced fresh parsley
Salt and pepper to taste
24 pieces julienned sun-dried tomatoes packed in oil

Halve eggs lengthwise. Remove yolks and force them through a fine sieve into a small nonreactive bowl. Stir in minced tomatoes, 4 tablespoons yogurt, capers, parsley, salt, and pepper. When well-combined, place in a pastry bag fitted with a large decorative tip and pipe into the egg-white cavities. Place a criss-cross of julienned tomato on top of each filled egg. Place remaining yogurt in a small pastry bag fitted with a small star tip. Pipe a yogurt star at either end of each filled egg between the crossed tomato strips. Serve immediately.

◆ TZATZIKI ◆

Makes 6 servings

6 pita breads
2 cups grated Kirby cucumber
1 teaspoon salt
1 1/4 cups plain regular, low-fat, or nonfat yogurt
2 cloves garlic, peeled and minced
1 tablespoon minced fresh parsley
1/2 cup chopped watercress

Preheat oven to 350°F.

Cut each pita into 6 pieces and pull apart. Place on an ungreased baking sheet in oven and bake for about 10 minutes, or until crisp. Remove from oven and set aside.

Place cucumbers in a sieve or colander, sprinkle with salt, and toss to combine. Place sieve over a bowl and allow to drain for at least 30 minutes. When well-drained, turn cucumbers out onto a clean kitchen towel. Pull up the corners and twist to press out all the liquid. Place in a serving bowl and stir in yogurt, garlic, and parsley. Cover and refrigerate for 20 minutes before serving. Garnish with chopped watercress and serve immediately with pita wedges.

◆ COCKTAIL KOFTAS ◆

Makes approximately 36 koftas

1 pound ground chicken or turkey
1/2 cup plain regular, low-fat, or nonfat yogurt
3 tablespoons minced garlic
1 tablespoon minced onion
1 tablespoon minced cilantro
2 teaspoons ground cumin
1 teaspoon ground coriander
1/4 teaspoon ground cinnamon
1/2 teaspoon cayenne pepper or to taste
Salt to taste
3 tablespoons peanut oil
One 1-inch piece cinnamon stick
4 whole cloves
3 whole cardamom pods
1 1/2 cups chopped red onion
1/2 cup peeled, seeded, and chopped very ripe tomato
1 tablespoon minced fresh ginger
1 teaspoon minced fresh green chile
1 teaspoon paprika
1 1/4 cups defatted unsalted chicken stock

Combine chicken, 3 tablespoons yogurt, 1/2 teaspoon garlic, minced onion, cilantro, 1 teaspoon cumin, 1/2 teaspoon coriander, ground cinnamon, 1/4 teaspoon cayenne, and salt, then form into approximately 36 small balls. Cover and set aside.

Heat oil in a large saucepan over medium–high heat. Add whole spices and meatballs, a few at a time. Stir to combine and fry until browned on all sides. Remove meatballs from pan and drain on paper towels. Add chopped onion to the pan. Lower heat to medium and fry, stirring frequently, until onions are well-browned but not burned, about 15 minutes. Add the remaining garlic, chopped tomato, ginger, chile, remaining ground spices, and paprika. Continue to fry, stirring frequently, for about 10 minutes or until mixture is nicely browned. Begin stirring in the remaining yogurt, a spoonful at a time, until it is well incorporated. Whisk in stock, then add meatballs. Lower heat, cover, and allow to just simmer for about 20 minutes or until the sauce has been absorbed by the meatballs, occasionally stirring gently.

Place toothpicks in meatballs (koftas) and serve. If necessary, pick the whole spices off the meatballs before serving.

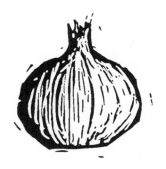

◆ BABA GHANOOJ ◆

Makes approximately 3 cups

One 1 1/2- to 2-pound eggplant
1/2 teaspoon salt
1/4 cup olive or canola oil
1/4 cup tahini (available in Middle Eastern or specialty
    food markets)
2 cloves garlic, peeled and chopped
1/4 cup fresh lemon juice
2 tablespoons minced fresh parsley
1 cup plain regular, low-fat, or nonfat yogurt
2 tablespoons toasted sesame seeds

Halve eggplant lengthwise and randomly pierce skin with a fork. Sprinkle cut side with salt and allow to drain on a wire rack for 1 hour. Pat dry.

Preheat oven to 400°F.

Place eggplant halves, cut side down, in a baking pan with sides. Add olive oil, place in oven, and bake for 25 minutes or until soft. Remove from oven and scoop out the pulp. Discard the skin.

Place pulp in a food processor fitted with the metal blade. Add tahini, garlic, lemon juice, and parsley. Process until smooth. Scrape from the food processor bowl into a nonreactive serving bowl. Stir in yogurt. Smooth top, and sprinkle with sesame seeds.

Serve at room temperature with raw or steamed vegetables, or as a dip with crackers.

EASY AND LOW-FAT
◆ HUMMUS ◆

Approximately 2 1/2 cups

One 19-ounce can chick-peas (garbanzos) or any other
    white bean, well drained
Juice of 1 lemon
5 cloves garlic, peeled and chopped
2 tablespoons chopped chives
1/2 teaspoon minced fresh hot chile or to taste
1/8 teaspoon ground cumin
1/2 cup plain regular, low-fat, or nonfat yogurt

Place all ingredients in a food processor fitted with the metal blade and process until smooth. Scrape into a bowl, cover, and refrigerate for at least 1 hour before serving.

Serve with chips, raw or steamed vegetables for dipping, or as an appetizer on a bed of chopped lettuce and tomato garnished with olives.

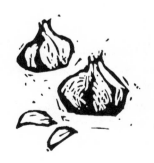

◆ CRUDITÉS WITH 3 DIPS ◆

Each dip makes approximately 3 cups

A crudité platter or basket is an easy, low-fat hors d'oeuvre that can be dressed up or down. It can be a fancy basket filled to the brim with beautiful baby and exotic vegetables or a few carrot and celery sticks on a picnic blanket. Either way calories are low and nutrition high, especially when accompanied by nonfat yogurt dips.

Any raw or al dente vegetable may become part of a crudité presentation. I often line a large basket with bunches of well-washed and dried chicory, escarole, or whatever lush, leafy green I can find. Then I build an arrangement of vegetables on and into the leafs, placing them in the most colorful pattern I can. Your imagination and the beauty of the vegetables are the only inspiration you will need. And the best thing of all is that when the party is over you can throw the entire crudité remains into a soup pot, add water, seasonings, and within minutes, a great vegetable soup is born. Puree it, serve either hot or cold with a dollop of leftover dip in the center, and you have a gourmet soup.

◆ Roasted Red Pepper Dip ◆

2 cups plain regular, low-fat, or nonfat yogurt

2 red bell peppers, roasted, peeled, stemmed, and seeded

2 cloves roasted garlic, peeled

1 teaspoon minced fresh basil

Salt and pepper to taste

◆ Curry Dip ◆

2 cups plain regular, low-fat, or nonfat yogurt
1/4 cup mayonnaise
1/4 cup minced scallions
1 tablespoon minced fresh mint
1 teaspoon curry powder
1/4 teaspoon ground cumin
Salt and pepper to taste

◆ Spicy Southwestern Dip ◆

2 cups plain regular, low-fat, or nonfat yogurt
1 ripe avocado, peeled and seeded
1 tablespoon minced fresh hot chile
Juice of 1 lime
2 tablespoons minced cilantro
1 clove garlic, peeled
Salt and pepper to taste

For each dip, combine all ingredients in a food processor fitted with the metal blade and process until smooth. Scrape into a small bowl, cover, and refrigerate until ready to serve.

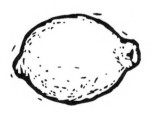

INDONESIAN SHRIMP BARBECUE
◆ WITH MANGO PUREE ◆

Makes 6 servings

1/2 cup plain regular, low-fat, or nonfat yogurt
1/4 cup chopped red bell pepper
1 fresh mildly hot red chile, chopped
2 cloves garlic, peeled and minced
2 tablespoons coconut milk (available in Asian or specialty
    food markets)
1 tablespoon fresh lemon juice
1 teaspoon light brown sugar
1/4 teaspoon shrimp paste (available in Asian or specialty
    food markets)
Salt to taste
18 jumbo shrimp, peeled and deveined
Mango Puree (recipe follows)

Combine all ingredients, except shrimp and mango puree. Add shrimp and cover and refrigerate for 1 hour.

Preheat broiler or grill.

Place 6 bamboo skewers in cold water to cover. When well-soaked, thread 3 shrimp on each skewer. Place under broiler or on grill for about 4 minutes, or until shrimp has curled and is cooked through, turning once. Serve immediately with mango puree.

Note: *You can also serve the shrimp individually placed on toothpicks, as hors d'oeuvres.*

◆ Mango Puree ◆

Makes approximately 1 cup

1 very ripe mango
1 tablespoon coconut milk (available in Asian or specialty
    food markets)
1 teaspoon fresh lime juice
1 teaspoon minced fresh mint

Peel and seed mango. Combine mango pulp with coconut milk and lime juice in a food processor fitted with the metal blade. Process until smooth. Stir in mint. Scrape into a small bowl, cover, and refrigerate until ready to use.

SOUPS, SALADS, AND
◆SIDE DISHES◆

Soups

Vichyssoise

Mixed Yogurt Gazpacho

Black Bean and Yogurt Soup

Cream of Vegetable-yogurt Soup

Southwestern Chowder

Roasted Eggplant Soup

Summer Cucumber Soup

Fruit Soup

Beet, Dill, and Yogurt Soup

Salads

Warm Red Potato Salad

New Wave Coleslaw

Bean Salad

Cucumber, Fennel, and Yogurt Cheese Salad

Wild Rice Salad

Mesclun Salad with Baby Beet Dressing

Composed Curried Chicken Salad

Roasted Vegetable Salad with Herbed Yogurt Dressing

Peanut Carrot Salad

Some Basic Salads: Egg, Chicken, Tuna

Side Dishes

Baked Stuffed Potatoes

Yogurt Roasted Potatoes

Roasted Vegetables with Spicy Yogurt

Wild Mushroom Ragout

Baked Sweet Potatoes

Vegetable Fritters

Yogurt Spiced Onion Rings

Custard Corn Pudding

Yogurt Noodles

Some Raitas
Cucumber-onion
Pineapple-mint
Carrot-cilantro
Tomato-parsley

◆ VICHYSSOISE ◆

Makes 6 servings

4 large Idaho potatoes
4 large leeks, white part only
1 tablespoon canola oil
3 cups defatted unsalted chicken stock
Salt and white pepper to taste
1 cup plain regular, low-fat, or nonfat yogurt
2 tablespoons minced fresh chives

Wash, peel, and dice potatoes. Place in cold water to cover and set aside.

Wash leeks, trim and use white part only. Cut into thin slices. Heat oil in a medium saucepan over medium heat, then add leeks and sauté for about 4 minutes or until just starting to soften.

Drain potatoes well and toss with sautéed leeks. Add stock, salt, and pepper and raise heat. Bring to a boil, then lower heat and simmer for 15 minutes or until potatoes are very soft. Immediately pour into a fine sieve or food mill and, using a spatula or wooden spoon, push potatoes and leeks through, catching all liquids and sieved vegetables in a storage container with a lid. Cool and refrigerate for at least 2 hours or until well chilled. Taste and adjust seasoning if necessary. Whisk in yogurt. If soup is too thick, add a bit of cold milk or stock. Pour into serving bowls and generously garnish with chopped chives.

Note: *To make this a nonmeat soup you may replace the stock with whole or skim milk.*

Do not use a food processor or blender to puree the potatoes and leeks as the high speed will make the soup very starchy.

MIXED YOGURT
◆ GAZPACHO ◆

Makes 6 servings

6 fresh tomatillos, husked, washed, and quartered
3 medium yellow tomatoes, peeled, cored, and seeded
1 yellow bell pepper, washed, cored, and seeded
1 seedless cucumber, peeled and cut into quarters
1 medium red onion, peeled and quartered
2 cloves garlic, peeled
1/2 jalapeño pepper, seeded, or to taste
1/4 cup cilantro leaves, washed and dried
1 very ripe avocado, peeled and seeded
1 cup plain regular, low-fat, or nonfat yogurt
1/2 cup champagne vinegar
2 tablespoons extra virgin olive oil
Salt and pepper to taste
Tabasco to taste
Fresh lime juice to taste
Spiced Yogurt (recipe follows)

One at a time coarsely chop tomatillos, tomatoes, bell pepper, and cucumber in a food processor fitted with the metal blade. Scrape each into a large mixing bowl as they are chopped. Then process onion, garlic, jalapeño, and cilantro until finely chopped. Scrape into the bowl with the chopped vegetables.

Next place avocado and yogurt in the food processor and process until smooth. Scrape into the bowl with the vegetables. Stir in vinegar, olive oil, salt, and pepper. If soup is too thick, thin with tomato or vegetable juice, or even cold water. Cover and refrigerate for at least 2 hours to allow flavors to develop. Taste and adjust seasoning with salt, pepper, Tabasco, and lime juice.

Pour into serving bowls and garnish with a dollop of spiced yogurt.

◆ Spiced Yogurt ◆

Makes 1/2 cup

1/2 cup plain regular, low-fat, or nonfat yogurt
1/2 teaspoon chili powder
1/4 teaspoon cayenne pepper
1/4 teaspoon freshly grated orange zest
Pinch ground cumin
Pinch salt

Whisk all ingredients together until well-combined. Cover and refrigerate until ready to use.

BLACK BEAN AND
◆ YOGURT SOUP ◆

Makes 6 servings

1 1/2 cups dried black beans, well rinsed
1 carrot, peeled and chopped
1/2 cup diced celery
1/2 cup diced onion
2 cloves garlic, peeled and minced
1 teaspoon minced fresh thyme
1/2 teaspoon minced fresh marjoram
1 1/4 cups ripe plum tomatoes, peeled, seeded, and diced
1 tablespoon minced fresh parsley
1 teaspoon fresh lemon juice
Salt and pepper to taste
1 cup plain regular, low-fat, or nonfat yogurt

Soak beans in cold water to cover, changing water at least three times in a 4-hour period. Drain well.

Place drained beans, carrot, celery, onion, garlic, and herbs in a deep saucepan with water to cover over high heat. Bring to a boil, then lower heat and simmer for 45 minutes or until beans are very soft. Place in a blender or food processor fitted with the metal blade and process until smooth, using whatever cooking liquid is necessary to make a thick soup.

Pour mixture into a clean saucepan. Stir in tomatoes, parsley, lemon juice, salt, and pepper and bring to a simmer over medium-high heat. Stir a small amount of soup into yogurt, then stir yogurt into the simmering soup. Stir until well-incorporated. Remove from heat and serve immediately.

Note: *This soup may be enriched with a ham bone or with chicken or meat stock in place of the water. It may also be served cold.*

CREAM OF VEGETABLE-
◆ YOGURT SOUP ◆

Makes 6 servings

1 tablespoon unsalted butter, margarine, or vegetable oil
1 tablespoon all-purpose flour
4 cups defatted unsalted chicken stock
1 pound peeled, chopped asparagus, carrots, squash or
　　tomatoes, or fresh shelled peas or lima beans, or
　　fresh corn kernels, or fresh leaf spinach,
　　well-trimmed and washed
1 cup chopped onion
1/4 cup chopped mushrooms
1 tablespoon minced fresh parsley
2 cups plain regular, low-fat, or nonfat yogurt
Tabasco to taste
Juice of 1/2 lime or to taste

Melt butter in a small saucepan over medium heat, then stir in flour. When well-blended, whisk in 1/2 cup stock. Stir until smooth and thick and set aside.

In a large saucepan, over medium high heat, combine 1/4 cup stock, vegetables, onion, mushrooms, and parsley. Cover and lower heat. Allow vegetables to sweat for about 5 minutes. Remove cover and add remaining stock. Raise heat and bring to a boil, then lower heat and simmer for about 15 minutes or until vegetables are soft. Pour soup into a blender and process until smooth, then pour into a clean saucepan. Whisk in flour mixture, place over medium-high heat. Bring to a simmer, then combine 1 cup hot soup with yogurt and whisk back into soup. Add Tabasco and lime juice and allow to just heat through. Serve hot, garnished with cooked pieces of whatever vegetables you have used, if desired.

Note: *To make this a nonmeat soup, the stock may be replaced with whole or skim milk or even water for much less fat and cholesterol as well as fewer calories.*

◆ SOUTHWESTERN CHOWDER ◆

Makes 6 servings

1 tablespoon canola oil
1 cup diced onion
1/4 cup diced celery
1/2 serrano chile, seeded and chopped, or to taste
2 cloves garlic, peeled and chopped
6 cups fresh corn kernels
1/2 cup diced Idaho potato
Salt to taste
4 cups defatted unsalted chicken stock
1/4 cup diced red bell pepper
1/4 cup diced green bell pepper
1 cup plain regular, low-fat, or nonfat yogurt, at room
    temperature
2 tablespoons minced cilantro
Cayenne pepper to taste

Heat oil in a heavy saucepan over medium heat, then add onion, celery, serrano, and garlic. Sauté for 4 minutes. Add half the corn, the potatoes, and salt and sauté for 3 minutes. Add stock and bring to a boil, then lower heat and simmer for 30 minutes or until vegetables are all very soft. Pour into a blender and process until quite smooth. Return to the saucepan over medium–high heat. Add remaining corn and bell peppers. Bring to a boil, then lower heat and simmer for 5 minutes. Stir in yogurt and cilantro and allow soup to just heat through. Do not boil. Serve immediately with a sprinkle of cayenne pepper on top.

◆ ROASTED EGGPLANT SOUP ◆

Makes 6 servings

One 1 1/2-pound eggplant
1/4 cup olive or vegetable oil
2 red bell peppers, washed, halved, cored, and seeded
2 ripe tomatoes, washed and cored
1 large red onion, washed and halved
6 cups unsalted vegetable stock
1 teaspoon minced fresh thyme
1 teaspoon minced fresh basil
Pinch saffron
Salt
Cayenne pepper to taste
1 1/2 cups plain regular, low-fat, or nonfat yogurt, at
    room temperature
1 cup croutons, warmed

Preheat oven to 375°F.

Wash and trim eggplant, cut in half and rub with some of the oil. Season with salt and pepper. Place cut side down on a nonstick baking sheet, put in oven, and roast for 20 minutes. Rub remaining vegetables with remaining oil and place on baking sheet with eggplant. Roast for an additional 25 minutes or until all vegetables are soft. Remove from oven and allow to cool until easy to handle. Peel eggplant, peppers, onion, and tomatoes. Place in a food processor fitted with the metal blade and process until smooth.

Scrape mixture into a medium saucepan. Stir in stock, thyme, basil, saffron, salt, and cayenne. Bring to a boil over high heat, then lower heat and simmer for 15 minutes. Whisk in yogurt and allow soup to just heat through. Do not boil!

Serve hot, topped with a few warm croutons.

◆ SUMMER CUCUMBER SOUP ◆

Makes 6 servings

6 cups shredded seedless cucumbers
1 teaspoon coarse salt
3 cups plain regular, low-fat, or nonfat yogurt
2 tablespoons buttermilk
1 tablespoon fresh orange juice
3 cloves garlic, peeled and finely minced
1 tablespoon minced fresh dill
1 tablespoon minced fresh mint
Freshly ground white pepper
Fresh herb sprigs or cucumber slices for garnish

Toss cucumbers with salt, then place in a sieve and allow to drain for 20 minutes. Put cucumbers in a clean kitchen towel and twist to press out all the liquid. Place drained cucumbers in a mixing bowl.

Combine yogurt, buttermilk, orange juice, garlic, dill, mint, and pepper, then pour over cucumbers and stir to combine. Cover and refrigerate for 30 minutes or until well-chilled. Serve cold garnished with fresh herb sprigs or cucumber slices.

Note: *This is a thick soup. If you prefer a thinner consistency, add more buttermilk, skim milk, or a little seltzer to thin it out. Don't add more orange juice as it will give the soup a definite citrus overtone.*

◆ FRUIT SOUP ◆

Makes 6 servings

3 cups chopped fresh berries, peaches, or nectarines
1 cup water, white wine, or champagne
2 cups fresh orange juice
1 tablespoon fresh lemon juice
1/4 cup sugar or to taste (see Note below)
Dash ground cumin
Dash ground nutmeg
2 cups plain or lemon regular, low-fat, or nonfat yogurt
2 tablespoons julienned mint leaves
1/2 cup whole berries or peach or nectarine slices

Combine chopped fruit, water, orange juice, lemon juice, sugar, and spices in a nonreactive saucepan over high heat. Bring to a boil, then lower heat and simmer for 10 minutes.

Pour mixture into a blender and process until smooth. (For berries, pour puree through a fine sieve and strain to eliminate any seeds.) Set aside to cool. When cool, combine with yogurt in a food processor fitted with the metal blade and process until smooth. Pour into serving bowls and garnish with julienned mint and whole berries or sliced peaches or nectarines.

Note: *The amount of sugar this soup requires will depend on the sweetness of the fruit. Remember, you want a tangy, refreshing soup, not a sweet dessert.*

BEET, DILL, AND
◆ YOGURT SOUP ◆

Makes 6 servings

1 1/2 pounds fresh beets
2 tablespoons raspberry vinegar
Salt to taste
2 tablespoons all-purpose flour
4 cups defatted unsalted chicken or beef stock
1 small onion, peeled and shredded
1 bay leaf
1 tablespoon light brown sugar
Freshly ground white pepper to taste
2 cups plain regular, low-fat, or nonfat yogurt
1/2 cup sour cream
2 tablespoons chopped fresh dill
6 lemon slices

Wash and trim beets, then using a food processor fitted with the shredding disk, shred them. Scrape into a nonreactive saucepan, add vinegar and salt, and toss to combine. Stir in flour until well-blended, adding a bit of water if necessary to eliminate any lumps. Add stock, onion, and bay leaf. Bring to a boil, then stir in sugar. Lower heat and simmer for 20 minutes. Remove from heat. Discard bay leaf and season to taste with salt and pepper.

Combine yogurt, sour cream, and dill. If soup is to be served cold, whisk yogurt mixture into soup. Pour into a nonreactive container, cover, and refrigerate for about 2 hours or until well-chilled.

If soup is to be served hot, have yogurt mixture at room temperature and stir it into soup after discarding bay leaf. Return to heat and allow soup to just heat through. Do not boil!

Either way, pour into serving bowls and garnish with a lemon slice.

Note: *To reduce cholesterol and calories, you may replace the stock with water and the sour cream with Imitation Sour Cream (page 9) or reduced-fat or reduced-calorie sour cream.*

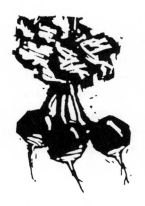

◆ WARM RED POTATO SALAD ◆

Makes 6 to 8 servings

2 pounds small red-skinned new potatoes
1/2 cup diced onion
Salt to taste
3/4 cup plain regular, low-fat, or nonfat yogurt
1/4 cup sour cream
4 scallions, trimmed and sliced
1 tablespoon well-drained bottled horseradish
3 tablespoons minced fresh dill
2 tablespoons crumbled cooked bacon
1 tablespoon raspberry vinegar
Freshly ground black pepper to taste

Scrub potatoes and cut into quarters. Place them in cold water to cover in a medium saucepan over high heat. Add onion and salt to taste. Bring to a boil, then lower heat and simmer for 15 minutes or until potatoes are just cooked. Remove from heat and drain well.

Place potatoes and onion bits in a serving bowl. Combine remaining ingredients and pour over potatoes. Toss well to coat potatoes, being careful not to break them up. Serve immediately.

◆ NEW WAVE COLESLAW ◆

Makes 6 to 8 servings

2 cups shredded green cabbage
2 cups shredded red cabbage
1 large carrot, peeled and shredded
1 Granny Smith apple, peeled, cored, and shredded
1/2 cup shredded onion
1/2 cup roasted unsalted sunflower seeds
1 cup plain nonfat yogurt
1/4 cup mayonnaise
3 tablespoons fresh orange juice
1 tablespoon sugar
1 tablespoon white vinegar
1/2 teaspoon Dijon-style mustard
One 1-inch piece fresh ginger, peeled
1/4 jalapeño pepper, optional

Combine cabbages, carrot, apple, onion, and sunflower seeds in a large bowl.

Whisk together yogurt, mayonnaise, orange juice, sugar, vinegar, and mustard.

Grate ginger into yogurt mixture.

Using a garlic press, carefully squeeze jalapeño into yogurt mixture. Stir to blend.

Pour dressing over cabbage mixture and toss to blend.

Cover and refrigerate for up to 3 hours before serving.

◆ BEAN SALAD ◆

Makes 6 servings

4 cups cooked, drained kidney beans
1/2 cup chopped fresh mint
1/2 cup chopped cilantro
1/4 cup chopped scallions
1 clove garlic, peeled and minced
1/3 cup plum preserves
2 tablespoons fruit vinegar
1 teaspoon brown sugar
3/4 cup plain regular, low-fat, or nonfat yogurt

Combine beans, herbs, scallions, and garlic in a mixing bowl and set aside.

Place plum preserves, vinegar, and sugar in a small saucepan over medium heat. Cook, stirring constantly, for about 4 minutes or until preserves have melted and sugar has dissolved. Remove from heat and pour into a blender. Process until smooth. Add yogurt and process to blend. Pour over bean mixture and toss to combine. Cover and allow to marinate for 2 hours. Serve at room temperature.

CUCUMBER, FENNEL, AND
◆ YOGURT CHEESE SALAD ◆

Makes 6 servings

2 pounds seedless cucumbers
1 fennel bulb
Juice of 1 orange
1 tablespoon white wine vinegar
1 teaspoon balsamic vinegar
1 small shallot, peeled and minced
1 teaspoon minced fresh mint
1/3 cup extra virgin olive oil
Salt and pepper to taste
1 cup Herb-flavored Yogurt Cheese (page 13)
12 whole mint leaves

Wash and dry cucumbers. Using a fork, score shallow lines down the entire length of each cucumber. Cut into thin slices. Place in a bowl, cover, and refrigerate for 30 minutes.

Trim the bulb end and outer leaves from fennel. Wash and dry well. Quarter the bulb, trim out the core, and slice lengthwise into very fine slices.

Combine orange juice, vinegars, shallot, minced mint, olive oil, salt, and pepper and set aside.

Layer the cucumber and fennel slices in an alternating pattern on a serving plate. Crumble yogurt cheese over top. Pour dressing over all and garnish with whole mint leaves. Serve immediately.

◆ WILD RICE SALAD ◆

Makes 6 servings

1 cup wild rice
Salt to taste
1 cup julienned snow peas
1/2 cup diced cooked carrots
1/2 cup chopped toasted hazelnuts
1/2 cup plain regular, low-fat, or nonfat yogurt
1/4 cup olive oil
1 tablespoon hazelnut oil
1/4 cup Japanese rice wine (available in Asian or specialty
   food markets)
1/4 teaspoon minced fresh ginger
1/2 teaspoon curry powder
Salt and pepper to taste

Rinse wild rice and place in cold water to cover for 30 minutes. Drain well. Place in a medium saucepan with 4 cups cold water and salt over high heat. Bring to a boil, then cover, lower heat, and simmer for about 35 minutes or until rice is tender but still chewy. Pour into a colander and allow to drain well.

Toss snow peas, carrots, and hazelnuts into rice.

Blend yogurt, oils, rice wine, ginger, curry powder, salt, and pepper, then pour over rice and stir to combine.

Serve as is or on a bed of California spinach or lettuce leaves.

MESCLUN SALAD WITH
◆ BABY BEET DRESSING ◆

Makes 6 servings

1/2 pound mesclun or a combination of garden-fresh
    baby lettuces
1 cup Yogurt Cheese, crumbled (page 8)
1/2 pound baby beets, cooked and peeled
1 tablespoon raspberry vinegar
2 teaspoons balsamic vinegar
4 tablespoons canola oil
1 tablespoon walnut oil
1 tablespoon minced fresh parsley
Salt and pepper to taste
1/2 cup toasted walnut pieces

Wash and dry greens and place on a serving platter. Sprinkle yogurt cheese over top.

Cut beets into fine julienne. Combine with vinegars, oils, parsley, salt, and pepper, then pour over greens and cheese. Sprinkle with toasted walnuts. Serve immediately.

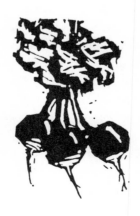

COMPOSED CURRIED CHICKEN
◆ SALAD ◆

Makes 6 servings

6 whole skinless, boneless chicken breasts
4 cups defatted unsalted chicken stock
Two 1-inch pieces fresh ginger, peeled
2 shallots, peeled and sliced
2 lemon wedges
Salt and pepper to taste
1 cup plain regular, low-fat, or nonfat yogurt
1/4 cup fresh orange juice
1 tablespoon wildflower honey
1 tablespoon light soy sauce
1 teaspoon curry powder or to taste
1/2 teaspoon grated fresh ginger
2 tablespoons minced cilantro
24 spears cooked asparagus
1 cup diced mango or papaya
3/4 cup chopped toasted cashews

Cut chicken breasts in half. Place in a shallow sauté pan with stock, ginger pieces, shallots, lemon, salt, and pepper. Add enough water to cover. Place over high heat and bring to a boil, then cover, lower heat and simmer for about 15 minutes or until chicken is cooked through. Remove chicken breasts from cooking liquid, place on a platter, and allow to cool. Discard cooking liquid or reserve for another use.

Combine yogurt, orange juice, honey, soy sauce, curry powder, and grated ginger, then stir in cilantro.

Cut chicken breasts crosswise on the diagonal into thin slices. Toss with yogurt dressing.

Fan 4 asparagus spears on each of six serving plates. Fan chicken slices on either side of asparagus. Place a mound of diced mango or papaya at the bottom. Sprinkle with toasted cashews and serve immediately.

ROASTED VEGETABLE SALAD WITH
◆ HERBED YOGURT DRESSING ◆

Makes 6 servings

6 to 8 cups sliced vegetables such as eggplant, any type
    squash, bell peppers, or beets
1/4 cup extra virgin olive oil
Grated zest and juice of 1 lemon
Salt and pepper to taste
1 cup plain regular, low-fat, or nonfat yogurt, at room
    temperature
1/3 cup herbed vinegar
2 tablespoons spicy mustard
1/4 cup chopped green olives
2 tablespoons minced fresh parsley
2 tablespoons minced fresh basil
1 teaspoon minced fresh marjoram
2 scallions, trimmed and chopped
Salt and pepper to taste

Preheat grill, or preheat oven to 375°F.

Toss vegetables with oil, lemon juice and zest, salt, and pepper. Place them on grill or in oven on a nonstick baking sheet. Roast for about 10 to 20 minutes, turning frequently, or until vegetables are just cooked through. Place on a serving platter.

Combine yogurt, vinegar, mustard, olives, herbs, scallions, salt, and pepper, then pour over warm vegetables. Serve immediately.

PEANUT CARROT
◆ SALAD ◆

Makes 6 servings

4 cups shredded carrots
1 cup diced apple
1 cup golden raisins (sultanas)
1/2 cup dry-roasted peanuts
3/4 cup lemon low-fat yogurt
1/2 teaspoon dry mustard
2 tablespoons fresh orange juice
1 tablespoon fresh lime juice
Cayenne pepper to taste
Salt to taste

Combine carrots, apples, raisins, and peanuts in a serving bowl.

Whisk together yogurt, mustard, citrus juices, cayenne, and salt, then pour over carrot mixture and toss to combine. Serve immediately, or cover and refrigerate until ready to serve.

SOME BASIC SALADS:
◆ EGG, CHICKEN, AND TUNA ◆

You can make any of our traditional salad sandwich fillings with yogurt mayonnaise in place of regular mayonnaise.

Here I give a basic recipe that I often vary for different flavors and caloric content. You can too!

◆ Yogurt Mayonnaise ◆

Makes approximately 3 cups

1/4 cup cider vinegar
1 tablespoon frozen apple juice concentrate, thawed
1/2 teaspoon salt
1 cup canola oil
1 cup plain regular, low-fat, or nonfat yogurt

OPTIONAL ADDITIONS
1 avocado, peeled and seeded
3 cloves garlic, peeled and minced
1/4 cup Dijon-style mustard
3 tablespoons minced fresh herbs
4 ounces soft cheese, such as blue, Roquefort, herbed or
    peppered goat cheeses

Combine vinegar, apple juice concentrate, and salt in a blender. Slowly add oil. When all oil is incorporated, scrape from the blender into a medium bowl.

Whisk in yogurt, then pour into a container with a lid and refrigerate until ready to use.

This dressing is delicious as is. However, if you wish additional body and flavor, blend in one, or any combination you like, of the optional ingredients after the oil has been incorporated.

◆ Egg Salad ◆

Makes 6 servings

8 hard-boiled eggs, peeled and chopped
1/4 cup diced celery
1/4 cup diced green bell pepper
1 teaspoon Dijon-style mustard
1/4 teaspoon celery seeds
3/4 cup Yogurt Mayonnaise (page 51)

Combine all ingredients. Use as a sandwich filling or salad, or cover and refrigerate until ready to serve.

◆ Chicken Salad ◆

Makes 6 servings

6 cups diced, cooked chicken breast
1/4 cup diced red onion
1/4 cup dried cherries, cranberries, blueberries, or
        currants, soaked in 2 tablespoons fresh orange juice
1 cup Yogurt Mayonnaise (page 51)

Combine all ingredients. Use as a sandwich filling or salad, or cover and refrigerate until ready to serve.

◆ Tuna Salad ◆

Makes 6 servings

**Two to three 6 1/8-ounce cans solid white tuna packed
 in water, well drained
1/2 cup diced celery
1 tablespoon pickle relish
1/2 to 3/4 cup Yogurt Mayonnaise (page 51)**

Combine all ingredients. Use as a sandwich filling or salad,
or cover and refrigerate until ready to serve.

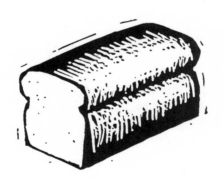

BAKED STUFFED
◆ POTATOES ◆

Serves 6

6 large Idaho potatoes
2 tablespoons canola oil
1 cup plain low-fat yogurt
2 tablespoons minced fresh chives
3 tablespoons grated Parmesan cheese
Salt and pepper to taste
1 teaspoon paprika

Preheat oven to 375°F.

Wash potatoes, pat dry, and pierce skins with a fork. Use 1 tablespoon canola oil to lightly coat their skins. Place in oven and bake for about 45 minutes or until centers of potatoes are cooked. Remove from oven and allow to cool slightly.

Slice potatoes in half lengthwise. Scrape out flesh into a mixing bowl and reserve skins. Use a fork to fluff potato. Add yogurt, chives, 2 tablespoons Parmesan, salt, and pepper. Whip together using a potato masher or whisk. Mound potato mixture back into reserved skins. Brush tops with remaining oil and sprinkle with remaining cheese and paprika. Place on a baking sheet and return to oven. Bake for about 5 minutes or until potatoes are hot and tops are a bit crisp. Serve hot.

YOGURT ROASTED
◆ POTATOES ◆

Makes 6 servings

6 to 8 large Idaho potatoes
1 cup plain regular, low-fat, or nonfat yogurt
1 teaspoon chili powder
Coarse salt to taste
Freshly ground black pepper to taste

Wash potatoes and dry well. Cut them lengthwise into 8 wedges and place in a shallow glass bowl. Add 2 tablespoons water. Cover with plastic wrap, poking 2 to 4 holes in it. Place in a microwave oven and microwave on high for approximately 12 minutes or until potatoes are cooked but still quite firm. Remove from microwave. Place potatoes on paper towels to drain well. Pat dry.

Preheat oven to 500°F.

Combine yogurt, chili powder, salt, and pepper and generously coat potato wedges with the mixture. Place on a baking sheet in the oven and bake for 10 to 15 minutes or until crisp and golden. Serve hot.

ROASTED VEGETABLES WITH
◆ SPICY YOGURT ◆

Makes 6 to 8 servings

2 cups sliced zucchini
2 cups sliced yellow squash
2 cups diced bell pepper
2 cups cooked pearl onions
1 cup diced artichoke hearts
2 tablespoons canola oil
Salt and pepper to taste
3/4 cup plain regular, low-fat, or nonfat yogurt, at room
    temperature
2 scallions, trimmed and chopped
1/2 serrano chile, minced fine
1 teaspoon cayenne pepper or to taste
Juice of 1/2 lemon

Preheat oven to 500°F.

Combine vegetables with oil, salt, and pepper. Place on a baking sheet in oven and bake for about 20 minutes or until cooked through and golden. Remove from oven and combine with remaining ingredients. Taste and adjust seasoning. Serve hot or at room temperature.

WILD MUSHROOM
◆ RAGOUT ◆

Makes 6 servings

5 large portobello mushrooms (or other large 3- to
    4-inch-diameter meaty mushrooms)
3 tablespoons extra virgin olive oil
1 tablespoon minced garlic
3 leeks, white part only, washed and thinly sliced
1 bulb fennel, trimmed and julienned
1 tablespoon minced fresh marjoram
Salt and pepper to taste
1 tablespoon balsamic vinegar
1/2 cup plain regular, low-fat, or nonfat yogurt, at room
    temperature

Trim stems from mushrooms and wipe clean. Slice stems
but leave caps whole. Set sliced stems aside.

Heat 2 tablespoons olive oil in heavy sauté pan over medium-high heat, then add mushrooms, top side down. Sprinkle 1
tablespoon olive oil and the garlic on the gills. Lower heat and cook
for 4 minutes. Turn caps over and cook for an additional 3 minutes
or until mushrooms are just cooked through. Remove mushrooms
from the pan and place in a bowl to drain. Keep warm.

Add sliced mushroom stems, leeks, fennel, and marjoram
to the pan. Sauté for about 5 minutes or until quite soft. Add salt
and pepper and sauté an additional 3 minutes. Slice the mushroom
caps and return them and any juices to the pan. Stir to combine
with the other vegetables. Stir in vinegar. When well-combined,
remove from heat. Stir in yogurt and serve warm.

◆ BAKED SWEET POTATOES ◆

Makes 6 servings

6 large sweet potatoes or yams
1 tablespoon canola oil
1/2 cup plain regular, low-fat, or nonfat yogurt
1/4 cup cooked brown rice
2 tablespoons minced dried apricots or prunes
1/2 teaspoon minced fresh sage
Salt and pepper to taste
2 tablespoons pure maple syrup

Preheat oven to 375°F.

Wash and dry potatoes. Pierce skins with a fork and lightly coat the skins with oil. Place them in oven and bake for about 45 minutes or until centers are cooked. Remove from oven and allow to cool slightly. Do not turn oven off.

Slice potatoes in half lengthwise. Scoop out flesh, leaving about a 1/8-inch border. Reserve skins.

Chop up flesh and gently toss with remaining ingredients (except for maple syrup). Mound filling back into potato skins. Place on a baking sheet and return to the hot oven to just heat through. Remove from oven.

Preheat broiler.

Drizzle top of each potato with a bit of maple syrup. Place potatoes under broiler for about 1 minute, to crisp tops. Serve immediately.

◆ VEGETABLE FRITTERS ◆

Makes 6 servings

1 cup plain regular, low-fat, or nonfat yogurt
1/2 cup skim milk
2 1/2 cups all-purpose flour
2 tablespoons baking powder
1 tablespoon minced shallots
2 tablespoons minced fresh parsley
1 teaspoon ground cumin
Tabasco sauce to taste
Salt and pepper to taste
6 cups shredded vegetables such as carrots, hard squash, or pumpkin
6 cups (approximately) vegetable oil

Whisk yogurt and skim milk together, then whisk in flour and baking powder. When well-blended, stir in shallots, parsley, cumin, Tabasco, salt, and pepper. Fold in shredded vegetables. Cover and let rest for 3 hours.

Heat oil in a deep-fat fryer or a deep saucepan to 360°F, then lower the batter into oil by heaping tablespoonsful. Fry for about 7–10 minutes or until golden. Do not crowd pan. Remove from oil and drain on paper towels. Continue frying until all the batter is used. Serve immediately with any of the yogurt sauces on pages 141–148, if desired.

YOGURT SPICED
◆ ONION RINGS ◆

Makes 6 servings

4 to 5 large sweet onions such as Vidalia
2 cups plain regular, low-fat, or nonfat yogurt
2 cups skim milk
1 tablespoon fresh lemon juice
3 cups all-purpose flour
3 tablespoons cornstarch
3 tablespoons fine cornmeal
1/3 cup chili powder
1 tablespoon hot paprika
1 teaspoon cayenne pepper or to taste
1 teaspoon ground cumin
1 teaspoon sugar
Salt to taste
Approximately 6 cups canola or other vegetable oil

Peel onions and cut crosswise into 1/4-inch thick slices. Pull slices apart into rings.

Whisk together yogurt, milk, and lemon juice in a nonreactive bowl, then add onion rings and toss to coat. Allow to marinate for 1 hour.

Combine flour, cornstarch, cornmeal, chili powder, paprika, cayenne, cumin, sugar, and salt.

Pour onions into a colander and allow to drain. Dredge rings, a few at a time, in the seasoned flour.

Heat oil in a deep-fat fryer or a deep saucepan to 360°F, then fry onion rings, a few at a time, for about 1 minute or until golden and crisp. Remove from oil and drain on paper towels. Serve hot.

◆ CUSTARD CORN PUDDING ◆

Makes 6 to 8 servings

3 large eggs
1 1/4 cups plain regular, low-fat, or nonfat yogurt, at
    room temperature
2 tablespoons melted unsalted butter
2 tablespoons all-purpose flour
1 tablespoon grated onion
1/2 teaspoon Tabasco
Salt and pepper to taste
2 cups cooked corn kernels
1/4 cup finely grated cheese (Parmesan or any low-fat
    hard cheese can be used)

Spray a 1 1/2-quart casserole with nonstick vegetable spray.
Preheat oven to 400°F.

Separate eggs. Beat whites until stiff but not dry.

Combine egg yolks, yogurt, butter, flour, onion, Tabasco,
salt, and pepper. Stir in corn, then fold in egg whites. Pour into the
prepared casserole. Sprinkle top with grated cheese. Place in oven
and bake for about 30 minutes or until golden and puffy. Remove
from oven and serve hot or at room temperature.

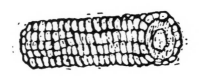

◆ YOGURT NOODLES ◆

Makes 6 servings

3/4 to 1 cup vegetable broth
1/2 cup chopped mushrooms
1/2 cup chopped onion
2 tablespoons minced fresh parsley
1 clove garlic, peeled and minced
Salt and pepper to taste
2 cups plain regular, low-fat, or nonfat yogurt
1 teaspoon poppy seeds
One 12-ounce package egg noodles

Heat 3/4 cup broth in a medium saucepan over medium-high heat. Add mushrooms, onion, 1 tablespoon parsley, and garlic. Bring to a boil, then lower heat and simmer for 10 minutes or until vegetables are very soft, adding additional broth if necessary to keep vegetables very moist. Add salt and pepper and remove from heat. Stir in yogurt and poppy seeds. Place over hot water or in a very low oven (200°F) to keep warm.

Cook noodles according to package directions. When cooked, drain well and pour into a bowl. Immediately pour yogurt sauce over them and toss to combine. Sprinkle with remaining minced parsley and serve immediately.

◆ SOME RAITAS ◆

Raitas are Indian relishes. They can be served as salads, condiments, dips, or sauces and can be either sweet or savory. These are just a sampling. Use your imagination to make raitas with what you have on hand. These all make 6 to 8 side-dish servings.

◆ Cucumber-onion Raita ◆

6 Kirby cucumbers
1 medium red onion
1 to 2 teaspoons coarse salt
1 cup plain regular, low-fat, or nonfat yogurt
1 tablespoon minced fresh dill
1 tablespoon pure maple syrup
Juice of 1 lime
1/2 teaspoon ground cumin
Cayenne pepper to taste

Wash cucumbers and cut crosswise into very thin slices. Peel and trim onion and cut crosswise into paper-thin slices. Combine cucumber, onion, and salt in a colander and place over a bowl to drain. Cover and refrigerate for 2 hours. Remove from the refrigerator and rinse under cold running water. Pat dry and set aside.

Combine yogurt, dill, syrup, lime juice, cumin, and cayenne in a nonreactive bowl. Add cucumber and onion and toss. Cover and refrigerate for 1 hour before serving. Taste and adjust seasoning, if necessary.

◆ Pineapple-mint Raita ◆

2 cups plain regular, low-fat, or nonfat yogurt
1 cup lemon regular, low-fat, or nonfat yogurt
1 cup diced fresh pineapple
3 tablespoons minced fresh mint
1/2 teaspoon minced serrano chile
Salt and pepper to taste

Combine yogurts, then stir in remaining ingredients. Cover and refrigerate until ready to serve.

◆ Carrot-cilantro Raita ◆

3 medium carrots, peeled and shredded
2 cups plain regular, low-fat, or nonfat yogurt
3 tablespoons chopped cilantro
2 tablespoons minced scallions
1/2 jalapeño pepper, seeded and minced, or to taste
1/2 teaspoon minced fresh ginger
Salt and pepper to taste

Place carrots in a steamer basket over boiling water and steam for 2 minutes or until crisp-tender. Refresh under cold running water. Drain dry.

Combine yogurt, cilantro, scallions, jalapeño, ginger, salt, and pepper, then toss in carrots. Cover and refrigerate until ready to serve.

◆ Tomato-parsley Raita ◆

2 cups diced tomatoes, well-drained
1 cup diced red onion
3 tablespoons minced fresh Italian (flat-leaf) parsley
1 tablespoon minced fresh basil
1 teaspoon minced fresh mint
Salt and pepper to taste
1 cup plain regular, low-fat, or nonfat yogurt

Combine all ingredients, cover, and refrigerate until ready to serve.

◆MAIN COURSES◆

Poultry

Tandoori Chicken

Chicken Enchiladas

Chicken Suprème with Artichoke Heart and Wild
Mushroom Sauce

Curried Chicken

Chicken Satay

Healthier "Fried" Chicken

Chicken Paprikas

Meat and Game

Shish Kebab

Roasted Leg of Lamb

Veal in a Pot

Calf's Liver à la Veneziana

Goulash

Meatballs in Yogurt Sauce

Sweet-and-sour Brisket

Fajitas with Tomato-onion Sauce

Rabbit Normandy

Seafood

Poached Salmon with Yogurt-dill Sauce

Grilled Yogurt-glazed Swordfish

Yogurt Herbed Steamed Fish

Grilled Halibut with Pineapple-yogurt Salsa

Sole en Papillote

Low-cal Shrimp Creole

Vegetable

Fettuccine, the Light Way

Yogurt Cheese–Stuffed Pasta Shells with Fresh Tomato-yogurt Sauce

Quiche

Cheddar Cheese, Yogurt, and Sun-dried Tomato Flan

Caponata Frittata

Asparagus Soufflé

Garbanzo Stew

◆ TANDOORI CHICKEN ◆

Makes 6 servings

3 pounds chicken pieces, skinned
2 teaspoons coarse salt
1/2 cup fresh lemon juice
1 cup plain regular, low-fat, or nonfat yogurt
1/2 cup chopped onion
3 cloves garlic, peeled and minced
1/2 fresh hot green chile
One 1-inch piece fresh ginger, peeled and chopped
1 teaspoon garam masala (available in Indian or specialty
    food markets)
2 tablespoons yellow food coloring mixed with 1
    tablespoon red food coloring, optional

Rinse chicken and pat dry. Make slits, on the diagonal, on the meatiest parts of chicken pieces. Lay pieces out in a single layer on a large platter or baking sheet. Sprinkle both sides with salt and lemon juice. Gently rub seasonings onto chicken. Cover and let rest for about 30 minutes.

Place remaining ingredients in a food processor fitted with the metal blade and process until smooth, then pour over chicken pieces. Cover and refrigerate for 24 hours, turning and basting occasionally.

Preheat oven to 500°F.

Remove chicken from the refrigerator and shake any excess marinade from each piece. Place on a wire rack on a baking sheet with sides. Place in oven and bake for about 15 to 20 minutes or until chicken is cooked through. Serve hot, with wedges of lemon or lime, if desired.

Note: *In India a tandoor is a deep oven made of clay and traditionally heated with wood or charcoal. The built-up heat is so intense* that whole chickens cook very quickly, sealing in juices and keeping the meat moist. The traditional bright orange color comes from food coloring, which I have given you the option of using.

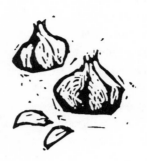

◆ CHICKEN ENCHILADAS ◆

Makes 6 servings

1 tablespoon canola oil
3 cups shredded, cooked chicken breast
2 cups shredded Monterey Jack, queso blanco, or other
  mild white cheese
1/2 cup chopped, peeled, and seeded roasted bell
  peppers
2 tablespoons minced cilantro
2 cups plain regular, low-fat, or nonfat yogurt, at room
  temperature
Salt and pepper to taste
12 flour tortillas
Enchilada Sauce (recipe follows)

Preheat oven to 350°F. Lightly oil a 12 × 14-inch baking dish and set aside.

Combine chicken, 1 1/4 cups cheese, bell peppers, and cilantro, then carefully fold in yogurt. Season with salt and pepper.

Place equal portions of filling down the center of each tortilla. Roll the sides of the tortilla in to the center to enclose filling. Place filled tortillas, seam side down, into the baking dish. Pour enchilada sauce over top. Place in oven and bake until filling is hot, about 15 minutes. Preheat broiler. Remove enchiladas from oven and sprinkle remaining cheese over top. Place under broiler for about 2 minutes or until cheese is melted and bubbling. Serve hot garnished with yogurt or Imitation Sour Cream (page 9), chopped cilantro, and hot sauce, if desired.

◆ Enchilada Sauce ◆

Makes approximately 4 cups

8 dried hot red chiles
2 cups diced onion
1 cup peeled, seeded, and diced ripe tomatoes
2 tablespoons minced garlic
1 tablespoon canola oil
1 tablespoon all-purpose flour
2 cups defatted unsalted chicken stock or water
Salt to taste

Soak chiles in cold water to cover until softened, about 20 minutes. Drain and remove stems and seeds.

Place chiles, onion, tomatoes, and garlic in a food processor fitted with the metal blade. Process until smooth.

Heat oil in a heavy sauté pan over medium-high heat, then pour in chile mixture. Lower heat and sauté for 5 minutes. Stir in flour until well-incorporated. Add stock and stir to combine. Cook, stirring frequently, for 15 minutes or until slightly thickened; add salt to taste. Use immediately, or cover and refrigerate for up to 1 week.

CHICKEN SUPRÈME WITH ARTICHOKE
◆ HEART AND WILD MUSHROOM SAUCE ◆

Makes 6 servings

6 chicken breasts, skinned, boned, and halved
2 cups plain regular, low-fat, or nonfat yogurt
1/4 cup fresh lemon juice
1 tablespoon Dijon-style mustard
1 teaspoon sweet paprika
Salt and pepper to taste
Artichoke Heart and Wild Mushroom Sauce (recipe
  follows)
1 tablespoon minced fresh parsley

Place chicken breasts in a nonreactive dish. Combine yogurt, lemon juice, mustard, paprika, salt, and pepper, then pour over chicken. Cover and refrigerate for 8 hours.

Preheat oven to 375°F.

Remove chicken from the refrigerator and shake off any excess marinade, then place in an ungreased baking dish. Put in oven and bake for about 25 minutes until cooked through. Remove from oven.

Place chicken breasts on a serving platter and pour artichoke heart and wild mushroom sauce over top. Sprinkle with parsley and serve immediately.

Artichoke Heart and
◆ Wild Mushroom Sauce ◆

Makes approximately 3 cups

1 tablespoon olive oil
2 cups sliced shiitake or other wild mushrooms
2 shallots, peeled and minced
2 cups defatted unsalted chicken stock
1 1/2 cups chopped cooked artichoke hearts
1 tablespoon fresh lemon juice
Salt and pepper to taste
1 cup plain regular, low-fat, or nonfat yogurt, at room
    temperature

Heat olive oil in a medium sauté pan over medium–high heat, then add mushrooms and shallots. Sauté for about 5 minutes or until mushrooms are wilted and shallots are translucent. Add stock. Raise heat and bring to a boil, then lower heat and simmer for 10 minutes or until liquid is reduced by half. Add artichoke hearts, lemon juice, salt, and pepper. Cook for 5 minutes. Remove about 1/4 cup liquid and stir into yogurt. Gently stir warmed yogurt, a bit at a time, back into sauce. Do not boil! When all the yogurt has been incorporated and sauce is warm, pour over chicken breasts, or place it in the top half of a double boiler over hot water to keep warm until ready to serve.

◆ CURRIED CHICKEN ◆

Makes 6 servings

2 tablespoons canola oil
1 cup chopped onion
3 cloves garlic, peeled and minced
1 tablespoon minced fresh ginger
1/2 fresh hot green chile or to taste
3 tablespoons Curry Spices or to taste (recipe follows)
2 cups peeled, seeded, and diced very ripe tomatoes
1 cup coconut milk (available in Asian or specialty food
   markets)
1 cup defatted unsalted chicken stock
1 1/2 pounds skinless, boneless chicken breasts
1 cup plain regular, low-fat, or nonfat yogurt, at room
   temperature
2 tablespoons minced cilantro
1/4 cup chopped toasted cashews

Heat 1 tablespoon oil in a heavy sauté pan over medium-high heat, then add onion, garlic, ginger, and chile. Lower heat and sauté for about 15 minutes or until onions are brown but not burned. Add spices and stir for 1 minute. Add tomatoes and stir to blend. Stir in coconut milk and stock, cover, and cook over low heat for 10 minutes.

Meantime, heat remaining oil in a sauté pan over medium-high heat, then add chicken pieces. Season with salt and pepper. Sauté for about 5 minutes or until chicken is firm and slightly browned. Remove from heat and drain on paper towels. When well-drained, scrape chicken into sauce. Cook for an additional 10 minutes or until chicken is cooked through.

Stir 1/4 cup sauce into yogurt. Gently stir warmed yogurt, a bit at a time, back into sauce. Stir in cilantro. Pour into a serving dish and garnish with chopped cashews. Serve with rice or noodles.

◆ Curry Spices ◆

Makes approximately 1 1/4 pounds

1 pound coriander seeds
1/4 pound cumin seeds
1 dried hot red chile, stem removed
1 tablespoon dried ginger
1 tablespoon sweet cumin seeds (available in Indian and
    specialty food markets)
1 tablespoon mustard seeds
1 tablespoon fenugreek
1 tablespoon cardamom seeds
One 2-inch stick cinnamon
8 black peppercorns
1 teaspoon whole cloves

Preheat oven to 250°F.

Place all ingredients on a baking sheet with sides and roast for 20 minutes. Remove from oven and immediately place in a blender or spice mill and process at high speed until all spices are ground very fine. Pour into a sterilized container with a lid and store in a cool, dark place for up to 3 months.

◆ CHICKEN SATAY ◆

Makes 6 servings

1 1/2 pounds skinless, boneless chicken breasts
1/2 cup plain regular, low-fat, or nonfat yogurt
1 1/2 cups Satay Sauce (recipe follows)

Cut chicken into 1-inch cubes. Place in a nonreactive bowl and add yogurt and 1/4 cup satay sauce. Toss to combine, cover, and refrigerate for 30 minutes.

Preheat grill or broiler.

Place 6 bamboo skewers in water to cover. When well-soaked, put equal portions of chicken on each skewer. Place on grill or under broiler and cook, turning occasionally, for about 4 minutes or until chicken is cooked through.

Heat remaining satay sauce and pass with chicken.

◆ Satay Sauce ◆

Makes about 2 cups

3/4 cup peanut butter
1/2 cup coconut milk (available in Asian or specialty food markets)
1/4 cup plain regular, low-fat, or nonfat yogurt
1 tablespoon light brown sugar
1/2 fresh hot green chile or to taste
2 tablespoons minced red onion
1 tablespoon minced garlic
1 tablespoon minced cilantro
1/2 teaspoon ground cumin
2 tablespoons fresh lime juice

Combine all ingredients in a food processor fitted with the metal blade. Process until smooth. Cover and refrigerate until ready to use. If mixture is too thick, thin with coconut milk, yogurt, or water.

◆ HEALTHIER "FRIED" CHICKEN ◆

Makes 6 servings

3 cups nonfat plain yogurt
1/2 cup buttermilk
2 tablespoons fresh lemon juice
2 cups all-purpose flour
1 cup plain bread crumbs
1 tablespoon freshly grated lemon zest
1 teaspoon minced fresh tarragon
Salt and pepper to taste
1 large frying chicken, cut into serving pieces, or chicken
    pieces as desired, washed and well-dried

Combine yogurt, buttermilk, and lemon juice in a shallow bowl and set aside.

Combine flour, bread crumbs, zest, tarragon, salt, and pepper in a brown paper or plastic bag.

Generously coat chicken pieces with yogurt mixture and toss in flour mixture, shaking to coat well. Set the floured chicken pieces on a platter being careful not to crowd them. Cover and refrigerate for 1 hour.

Preheat oven to 400°F.

Generously coat a baking sheet with sides with nonstick vegetable spray, or use a nonstick sheet pan. Lay chicken pieces on the prepared pan being careful not to crowd them. Use two pans if necessary. Place in oven and bake for 45 minutes, turning once, until chicken is golden brown and crisp. Serve hot or at room temperature.

◆ CHICKEN PAPRIKAS ◆

Makes 6 servings

5 pounds chicken pieces or cut-up whole chicken
1/2 cup all-purpose flour
Salt and pepper to taste
2 tablespoons fine Hungarian paprika
2 tablespoons canola oil
3 cups diced onion
1 cup defatted unsalted chicken stock
1 cup plain regular, low-fat, or nonfat yogurt, at room
    temperature
1/2 cup regular, low-fat, or nonfat sour cream

Combine chicken, flour, salt, pepper, and paprika, tossing to coat.

Heat oil in a heavy sauté pan over medium-high heat, then brown chicken pieces, a few at a time, for about 4 minutes or until well-browned on all sides. Drain on paper towels. When all the chicken is browned, add onions to the pan and sauté for 5 minutes. Add the stock, raise heat to high, and bring to a boil, scraping the brown bits from the bottom of the pan as you go. Add chicken and lower heat to a simmer. Cover and simmer for 1 hour or until chicken is very tender. Remove from heat. Combine yogurt and sour cream. Stir into chicken and serve immediately with noodles, if desired.

◆ SHISH KEBAB ◆

Makes 6 servings

1 1/4 pounds boneless lamb
2 cups plain regular, low-fat, or nonfat yogurt
Juice of 1 lemon
3 cloves garlic, peeled and minced
1 teaspoon minced fresh oregano
1 teaspoon minced fresh thyme
Coarse salt to taste
Freshly ground black pepper to taste
1 red bell pepper
1 green bell pepper
1 pint basket cherry tomatoes
6 to 12 small white mushrooms

Remove any fat from lamb and cut into 1-inch cubes. Place in a nonreactive container.

Combine yogurt, lemon juice, garlic, oregano, thyme, salt, and pepper, then pour over lamb cubes and toss to coat well. Cover and refrigerate for 6 hours, turning occasionally.

Wash and dry bell peppers. Core, seed, and devein them, then cut into 1-inch squares.

Wash and dry tomatoes.

Wipe mushrooms clean and remove stems.

Remove lamb from marinade, shaking off any excess. Toss vegetables with remaining marinade to just coat.

Preheat grill or broiler.

Thread lamb and vegetables on metal skewers in an attractive pattern. Place skewers on grill or under broiler. Grill, turning occasionally, about 15 to 20 minutes or until meat is cooked and vegetables are softened. Serve hot with rice, if desired.

Note: *You may replace the lamb with any other meat or poultry and add other vegetables such as squash, pearl onions, or eggplant.*

◆ ROASTED LEG OF LAMB ◆

Serves 6–8

One 4 1/2- to 5-pound leg of lamb, trimmed of silver skin
    and excess fat
15 cloves garlic, peeled
2 cups plain regular, low-fat, or nonfat yogurt
Juice of 1 lemon
1 tablespoon celery seeds
1 tablespoon turmeric
Coarse salt to taste
Cracked black pepper to taste

Using the point of a paring knife, make 15 small slits in lamb. Insert a garlic clove into each slit. Place lamb in a shallow, nonreactive pan. Combine yogurt, lemon juice, celery seeds, and turmeric, then pour over lamb. Cover and refrigerate for 24 hours, turning occasionally.

Preheat oven to 500°F.

Place lamb on a wire rack in a roasting pan. Generously season with salt and pepper. Place in oven and roast for 30 minutes. Lower heat to 375°F and roast for approximately 70 minutes (for rare) or until an instant-read thermometer inserted into the meatiest part reads 145°F for rare, 160°F for medium, or 175°F for well-done.

Remove from oven and allow to rest for about 10 minutes before carving.

◆ VEAL IN A POT ◆

Makes 6 servings

One 3-pound, 1-inch-thick veal steak
1/2 cup all-purpose flour
1/2 teaspoon paprika
1/4 teaspoon dry mustard
Salt and pepper to taste
1 tablespoon canola oil
12 pearl onions
2 cups diced carrots
1 cup diced celery
1 cup sliced mushrooms
3 cups skim milk, vegetable stock, or water
1/2 cup plain whole milk yogurt, at room temperature

Trim any excess fat from veal steak. Combine flour, paprika, mustard, salt, and pepper and dredge veal in it. Lightly pound flour into meat with a mallet or the edge of a heavy plate.

Heat oil in a deep, heavy sauté pan over medium-high heat, then brown veal steak for about 3 minutes per side or until well-seared. Remove meat and carefully wipe excess fat from the pan. Return meat to the pan and cover with vegetables and milk. Place over medium heat and bring to a simmer. Cover and simmer for about 45 minutes, or until meat is very tender. Remove from heat and stir in yogurt. Serve immediately with noodles, if desired.

◆ CALF'S LIVER À LA VENEZIANA ◆

Makes 6 servings

2 tablespoons olive oil
1 cup thinly sliced sweet onion such as Vidalia
1 tablespoon chopped fresh sage
1 teaspoon freshly grated lemon zest
1/4 cup dry white wine
1 1/2 pounds calf's liver, thinly sliced
1 tablespoon unsalted butter
3 tablespoons extra fine flour such as Wondra
Salt and pepper to taste
1 cup plain regular, low-fat, or nonfat yogurt, at room
    temperature

Heat 1 tablespoon olive oil in a large sauté pan over medium-high heat, then stir in onions. Lower heat and sauté for about 20 minutes or until onions are quite brown and very soft. Stir in sage, zest, and wine and cook for an additional 3 minutes. Remove from heat and set aside.

Trim liver of any thin skin and gristle and slice thinly. Lightly coat the slices with flour, salt, and pepper. Heat remaining oil and butter in a large sauté pan over medium-high heat, then add liver slices and fry for about 1 minute per side or until liver has crisped but is still rare. Do not crowd pan. Cook in batches if necessary, keeping liver warm as you fry.

When all liver is fried, add onions to the pan and cook, scraping up any brown bits from the bottom of the pan. Remove from heat and stir in yogurt. Place liver on a serving plate and pour onions over the top. Serve immediately.

◆ GOULASH ◆

Makes 6 servings

2 pounds lean pork, cut into 2-inch cubes
1/2 cup all-purpose flour
Salt and pepper to taste
1 tablespoon hot Hungarian paprika
2 tablespoons canola oil
2 cups diced onion
1 1/2 cups sliced mushrooms
1 cup defatted unsalted chicken stock
1 cup chopped canned plum tomatoes, well-drained
1 tablespoon cornstarch
1 1/4 cups plain regular, low-fat, or nonfat yogurt, at
    room temperature
1/2 cup sour cream
2 tablespoons minced fresh parsley

Combine pork, flour, salt, pepper, and paprika, tossing to coat cubes of pork.

Heat oil in a heavy Dutch oven over medium-high heat, then sear pork, a few pieces at a time, for about 4 minutes or until well-browned on all sides. Remove from pan and drain well on paper towels. Add onions to the pan and sauté for 2 minutes, then add mushrooms and sauté for an additional 3 minutes. Add stock. Raise heat, bring to a boil, scraping brown bits from the bottom of the pan as you stir, then add pork and tomatoes. Lower heat and simmer for 1 hour or until pork is very tender. Remove from heat. Dissolve cornstarch in 1 tablespoon cold water, then stir into yogurt. Combine yogurt and sour cream, then stir into goulash along with parsley. Serve immediately with noodles or rice, if desired.

MEATBALLS IN
◆ YOGURT SAUCE ◆

Makes 6 servings

3/4 pound lean ground beef
3/4 pound lean ground veal or pork
1 cup extra fine bread crumbs
1 large egg white
1/2 cup minced onion
3 tablespoons minced fresh parsley
Freshly ground nutmeg to taste
Salt and pepper to taste
2 to 3 tablespoons vegetable oil
3 tablespoons all-purpose flour
2 cups defatted unsalted beef stock
1 teaspoon cornstarch
1 1/4 cups plain regular, low-fat, or nonfat yogurt, at
    room temperature

Combine meat, bread crumbs, egg white, onion, 1 tablespoon parsley, nutmeg, salt, and pepper and form into small meatballs. Heat oil in a sauté pan over medium heat, then add meatballs, a few at a time, and fry until well-browned. Remove to paper towels to drain. Continue to fry until all meatballs are browned. Stir flour into fat remaining in the pan. When flour has been absorbed, add stock, whisking as you pour. Bring to a boil, whisking constantly, then return meatballs to the sauce. Lower heat and cook for 20 minutes.

Dissolve cornstarch in 1 tablespoon cold water and stir into yogurt, then stir into meatballs. Continue to cook until sauce is hot. Do not boil! Stir in remaining parsley. Serve hot with new potatoes, noodles, or rice, if desired.

SWEET-AND-SOUR
◆ BRISKET ◆

Makes 6 servings

1 tablespoon vegetable oil
8 large onions, peeled and thinly sliced
2 pounds beef brisket, well-trimmed
salt and pepper to taste
2 bay leaves
2 tablespoons frozen apple juice concentrate, thawed
1/4 cup cold water
1 cup well-drained diced canned plum tomatoes
1/4 cup raisins
3 gingersnaps, well-crumbled
1/4 cup brown sugar
Juice of 1 lemon
3/4 cup plain regular, low-fat, or nonfat yogurt, at room
    temperature
2 tablespoons minced fresh parsley

Heat oil in a Dutch oven over medium heat, then add onions. Lower heat and sauté for about 15 minutes or until onions are well-browned but not burned. Rub meat with salt and pepper. Place on top of onions and sear for about 4 minutes, or until all sides are brown. Add bay leaves, apple juice concentrate, and water. Lower heat and cover tightly. Allow to simmer for about 2 hours or until meat is tender. You may have to add a bit of water to keep meat from sticking. Uncover and stir in tomatoes, raisins, gingersnaps, brown sugar, and lemon juice. Continue to simmer for about 30 minutes or until meat is very tender and gravy is thick. Remove meat and place on a platter. Remove bay leaves. Stir a bit of hot gravy into yogurt, then stir yogurt, a bit at a time, back into gravy. Taste and adjust seasoning.

Slice meat on the cross grain into very thin slices. Generously coat with gravy. Garnish with minced parsley and serve immediately.

FAJITAS WITH
◆ TOMATO-ONION SAUCE ◆

Makes 6 servings

12 flour tortillas
2 ripe avocados
Juice of 1 lime
2 tablespoons minced cilantro
Salt and pepper to taste
1 1/2 to 2 pounds flank steak
1 teaspoon cayenne pepper or to taste
Tomato-onion Sauce (recipe follows)
1 cup plain regular, low-fat, or nonfat yogurt

Preheat oven to 350°F. Wrap tortillas in aluminum foil and place in oven for 10 minutes to heat through. Remove and keep warm.

Peel and chop avocados. Combine with the lime juice, cilantro, salt, and pepper and set aside.

Preheat grill or broiler.

Rub steak with salt and cayenne. Place on grill or under broiler and grill for about 4 minutes per side (for rare) or until steak is cooked to desired degree of doneness. Remove from grill and allow to rest for 5 minutes. Cut steak diagonally on the cross grain into very thin slices.

Place equal portions of steak down the center of each warm tortilla. Add equal portions of avocado, then top with equal portions of tomato–onion sauce and yogurt. Fold sides of the tortilla in to the center to enclose filling. Serve immediately, two per person.

Tomato-onion
◆ Sauce ◆

Makes about 4 cups

3 tablespoons defatted unsalted chicken stock
2 cups diced red onion
2 tablespoons minced garlic
1 fresh hot green chile, stemmed and chopped, or to
   taste
2 cups well-drained diced canned plum tomatoes
One 4-ounce can diced green chiles, well-drained
1 tablespoon chili powder
1 teaspoon minced fresh oregano
1/2 teaspoon ground cumin
Salt and pepper to taste

Heat stock in a medium sauté pan over medium-high heat, then add onion, garlic, and fresh chile. Cover and allow to cook for 5 minutes. Uncover, add tomatoes, chopped green chiles, chili powder, oregano, cumin, salt, and pepper. Cook for 10 minutes. Remove from heat and allow to sit for 15 minutes before using, or cool slightly, cover, and refrigerate for up to 1 week.

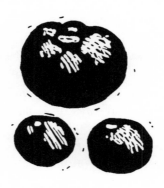

◆ RABBIT NORMANDY ◆

Makes 6 servings

2 cups apple cider
2 cups defatted unsalted chicken stock
1 cup dry white wine
6 rabbit loins
Salt and pepper to taste
2 tablespoons canola oil
1 tablespoon unsalted butter or margarine
2 cups pared, cored, and diced Granny Smith apples
1/4 cup minced shallots
1 stalk celery, washed, trimmed, and minced
4 teaspoons minced fresh tarragon
1 teaspoon minced fresh parsley
1 cup plain regular, low-fat, or nonfat yogurt, at room
   temperature
1/2 cup toasted walnut pieces

Place apple cider, stock, and wine in a heavy saucepan over high heat. Bring to a boil, then lower heat and simmer for 30 minutes or until reduced by half. Set aside.

Preheat oven to 350°F.

Trim loins of all fat and silver skin. Season with salt and pepper. Heat oil in a large, ovenproof sauté pan over medium-high heat, then add loins and sear for about 4 minutes or until all sides are brown. Place pan in oven and roast loins for 12 minutes or until meat is just cooked. Do not overcook. Remove from oven and place loins on a platter. Keep warm.

Return the sauté pan to medium-high heat and add butter. When butter has melted add apples, shallots, celery, tarragon, and parsley. Sauté for about 5 minutes or until apples begin to soften. Add the reduced cider-stock mixture and bring to a boil, then lower heat and simmer for 5 minutes. Stir 1/2 cup hot apple mixture into yogurt, then whisk back into apple mixture. Cook, but do not boil, until sauce is hot.

Slice loins on the diagonal. Place 1 loin on each of six dinner plates. Generously coat with apple mixture. Garnish with toasted walnuts and serve immediately.

POACHED SALMON WITH
◆ YOGURT-DILL SAUCE ◆

Makes 6 servings

1 1/2 cups minced onion
Juice of 2 limes
2 tablespoons fresh orange juice
2 tablespoons minced fresh parsley
1 teaspoon minced fresh dill
1 teaspoon minced fresh marjoram
Six 6-ounce salmon steaks
Yogurt-dill Sauce (recipe follows)

Preheat oven to 400°F.

Combine onion, lime and orange juices, and herbs, then scrape into a glass baking dish large enough to hold the fish in a single layer. Lay fish on top of onion mixture. Cover tightly with aluminum foil. Place in oven and bake for about 15 minutes or until just cooked. Remove from oven and uncover. Scrape onion bits off the bottom of each steak and discard; place steaks on a serving platter. Coat each steak with yogurt-dill sauce. Serve individually, passing remaining sauce on the side.

Note: *This is also terrific cold. Cover and refrigerate cooked salmon steaks for about 3 hours to chill well before serving.*

◆ Yogurt-dill Sauce ◆

Makes about 1 3/4 cups

1 1/2 cups plain regular, low-fat, or nonfat yogurt
1 teaspoon Dijon-style mustard
3 tablespoons minced fresh dill
2 teaspoons grated onion
1 teaspoon freshly grated orange zest
Salt and black pepper to taste
Freshly ground white pepper to taste

Combine all ingredients, cover, and chill for at least 3 hours.

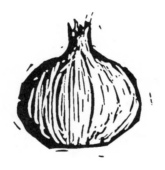

GRILLED YOGURT-GLAZED
◆ SWORDFISH ◆

Makes 6 servings

1 1/2 cups plain regular, low-fat, or nonfat yogurt
1/2 cup mayonnaise
1 cup loosely packed watercress leaves
1/4 cup chopped fresh dill
2 cloves garlic, peeled and chopped
Salt and pepper to taste
Six 6-ounce, 1-inch-thick swordfish steaks

Place yogurt in a fine sieve and allow to drain for 15 minutes. Combine drained yogurt, mayonnaise, watercress, dill, garlic, salt, and pepper in a food processor fitted with the metal blade.

Preheat grill.

Using half the yogurt mixture, spread equal portions on one side of each of the swordfish steaks. Place fish, yogurt side down, on grill and grill for 6 minutes. Just before turning, use remaining yogurt mixture to coat the top sides of the fish. Turn and grill for an additional 6 minutes or until swordfish is cooked through. Serve immediately.

YOGURT HERBED STEAMED
◆ FISH ◆

Makes 6 servings

2 cups plain regular, low-fat, or nonfat yogurt
1/2 cup chopped fresh chives
1/2 cup chopped spinach
2 tablespoons minced fresh parsley
1 tablespoon minced shallot
1 tablespoon fresh lemon juice
Salt and pepper to taste
One 5- to 6-pound whole fish such as sea bass or red
  snapper
6 to 8 large romaine lettuce leaves, washed

Combine yogurt, chives, spinach, parsley, shallot, lemon juice, salt, and pepper in a food processor fitted with the metal blade. Generously coat fish with it and place about 1/2 cup in the cavity as well. Reserve any remaining sauce.

Place lettuce on the rack of fish poacher or steamer. Add enough water to barely cover bottom, but do not allow it to touch the rack. Bring water to a boil over high heat, then place fish on its side on the rack. Cover tightly and steam for about 15 minutes or until fish is just cooked through. Remove rack from poacher. Carefully roll fish off rack onto a serving platter. Serve hot or chilled with remaining sauce.

GRILLED HALIBUT WITH
◆ PINEAPPLE-YOGURT SALSA ◆

Makes 6 servings

1 small pineapple, peeled and cored
1/2 cup lemon or plain low-fat yogurt
2 tablespoons minced cilantro
1 shallot, peeled and minced
1/2 teaspoon minced fresh ginger
1/2 teaspoon minced fresh hot green chile
Juice of 1 lime
Salt and pepper to taste
Six 6-ounce halibut steaks

Cut pineapple into chunks. Place in a food processor fitted with the metal blade and process until coarsely chopped, then put it in a fine sieve and allow to drain over a bowl. When well-drained, place pineapple in a nonreactive bowl. Reserve juice. Combine pineapple with yogurt, cilantro, shallot, ginger, chile, lime juice, salt, and pepper. Set aside.

Preheat grill.

Rub halibut steaks with the reserved pineapple juice, salt, and pepper. Place on grill for about 5 minutes per side, or until fish is just cooked through. Serve hot with some of the pineapple-yogurt salsa spooned over the top. Pass remaining salsa.

◆ SOLE EN PAPILLOTE ◆

Makes 6 servings

Six 12 × 15-inch pieces parchment paper
Six 6-ounce, 1/4-inch-thick sole fillets
Salt and pepper to taste
1 cup Herb-flavored Yogurt Cheese (page 13)
1/2 cup diced yellow bell pepper
1/4 cup diced red onion
2 tablespoons minced fresh parsley
6 lime wedges

Preheat oven to 425°F.

Fold parchment paper in half lengthwise. Cut each folded piece into a half heart about 7 inches longer and 3 inches wider than the fillets. Open each folded heart and lay it out flat. Place one fish filet on the right half of each heart. Season with salt and pepper.

Crumble yogurt cheese or cut into small bits. Combine with bell pepper, onion, and parsley, then place equal portions on top of each fillet. Fold the other heart half up and over the cheese-topped fillet, lining up the edges of the paper. Working from the top, seal the packet by folding in the edges, a small section at a time. You will have to fold over twice to ensure a tight seal. When you get to the bottom point, twist to hold the packet together.

Place completed packets in a single layer in a shallow baking pan. Place in oven and bake for about 12 minutes or until fish is just cooked.

Remove from oven and allow to rest for 1 minute.

Place on a serving platter. Cut an opening in the top of each packet to allow steam to escape. Pull rolled paper apart and serve hot with a wedge of lime.

LOW-CAL SHRIMP
◆ CREOLE ◆

Makes 6 servings

3 tablespoons water
2 cups diced onion
1 tablespoon minced garlic
1 cup diced red bell pepper
1 cup diced green bell pepper
1/2 cup dry white wine
2 bay leaves
1 teaspoon paprika
1 teaspoon minced fresh oregano
1 teaspoon minced fresh thyme
2 cups diced canned plum tomatoes
Salt and pepper to taste
2 pounds shelled and deveined shrimp
1 teaspoon cornstarch dissolved in 1 tablespoon cold
    water
1 cup plain regular, low-fat, or nonfat yogurt, at room
    temperature
6 to 8 cups hot cooked rice
3 tablespoons minced fresh parsley

Place water, onion, and garlic in a Dutch oven over medium-high heat. Bring to a boil, then lower heat, cover, and
simmer 5 minutes. Add peppers and cook, stirring frequently, for
5 minutes. Add the wine, bay leaves, paprika, oregano, and thyme.
Cook for 5 minutes. Add tomatoes, salt, and pepper. Cook for 5
minutes more. Add shrimp and cook for another 5 minutes. Stir in
cornstarch mixture and cook, stirring constantly, for 3 minutes. Stir
in yogurt and cook for 1 minute or until yogurt is well-incorporated and sauce is hot.

Place rice on a serving platter. Pour shrimp over it, sprinkle with parsley, and serve immediately.

FETTUCCINE, ◆ THE LIGHT WAY ◆

Makes 6 servings

3 tablespoons defatted unsalted chicken stock
1 cup diced wild mushrooms
2 tablespoons minced onion
1 cup grated Parmesan cheese
2/3 cup plain regular, low-fat, or nonfat yogurt, at room temperature
Freshly ground white pepper to taste
One 12-ounce package spinach fettuccine
1 tablespoon minced Italian (flat-leaf) parsley

Heat stock in a medium saucepan over medium–high heat, then add mushrooms and onion. Cover and cook for 5 minutes or until mushrooms are very soft. Whisk in cheese and yogurt. Lower heat and cook, stirring constantly, until sauce is hot. Do not boil! Season with pepper. Keep warm over hot water until ready to serve.

Cook fettuccine according to package directions. Drain well and put in a serving bowl. Pour sauce over top and toss to combine. Sprinkle with parsley and serve immediately.

YOGURT CHEESE–STUFFED PASTA SHELLS WITH FRESH
◆ TOMATO-YOGURT SAUCE ◆

Serves 6

24 jumbo pasta shells
One 10-ounce package frozen chopped spinach, thawed
    and well-drained
2 large eggs
2 large egg whites
1 1/2 cups Yogurt Cheese (page 8)
1 1/2 cups shredded mozzarella cheese
Freshly ground nutmeg to taste
Fresh Tomato-yogurt Sauce (recipe follows)
1/4 cup grated Parmesan cheese, optional

Cook shells according to package directions. Drain well.
Preheat oven to 350°F.

Beat spinach, eggs and egg whites, cheeses, and nutmeg
together, then scoop an equal portion into each well–drained shell.
Place shells, in a single layer, in a greased shallow baking dish. You
may need two dishes. Spoon a bit of the tomato-yogurt sauce over
each shell. Cover tightly and place in oven. Bake for 20 minutes or
until filling is hot. Remove from oven, uncover, and spoon remaining sauce over all. Sprinkle with grated Parmesan and serve
immediately.

◆ Fresh Tomato-yogurt Sauce ◆

Makes approximately 5 cups

1 cup light cream cheese
1 cup plain regular, low-fat, or nonfat yogurt
1 cup skim milk
2 tablespoons all-purpose flour
Salt and pepper to taste
2 cups peeled, seeded, and diced very ripe tomatoes
2 tablespoons minced fresh basil

Combine cream cheese, yogurt, and milk in a blender. Pour into a small saucepan over low heat. Whisk in flour, salt, and pepper, then stir in tomatoes and basil. Keep warm over hot water until ready to serve. Do not allow sauce to boil.

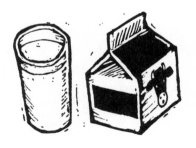

◆ QUICHE ◆

Makes 6 servings

2 cups grated Gruyère or other cheese (low-fat may be
   used)
1/2 cup crumbled cooked bacon
1 unbaked 9-inch pie shell
4 large eggs
1 1/4 cups plain regular, low-fat, or nonfat yogurt
1 tablespoon all-purpose flour
Tabasco to taste
Freshly ground nutmeg to taste
2 tablespoons grated Parmesan cheese

Preheat oven to 400°F.

Combine cheese and bacon and cover the bottom of the
pie shell with it.

Combine eggs, yogurt, flour, Tabasco, and nutmeg in a
blender, then pour over cheese and bacon. Use your fingertips to
gently mix cheese and bacon into egg mixture. Sprinkle top with
Parmesan cheese. Place on a baking sheet in oven and bake for 15
minutes. Lower heat to 350°F and bake for about 20 minutes more
or until center is set and crust is golden. Remove from oven and
cool on a wire rack for 10 minutes before serving.

Note: *You may use the basic recipe, with or without the bacon,
to make any vegetable, meat, or seafood quiche. It is best to use cooked,
well-drained ingredients when making a flavored quiche.*

CHEDDAR CHEESE, YOGURT, AND
◆ SUN-DRIED TOMATO FLAN ◆

Makes 6 servings

4 large eggs
1 1/2 cups plain regular, low-fat, or nonfat yogurt, at
    room temperature
1/4 cup water
1/2 cup all-purpose flour
1 cup shredded cheddar cheese
1/4 cup diced sun-dried tomatoes packed in oil,
    well-drained
1 tablespoon minced onion
1 teaspoon minced fresh basil
1 teaspoon minced fresh parsley
Salt and pepper to taste

Preheat oven to 425°F.

Spray a 9-inch pie dish with nonstick vegetable spray. Set aside.

Whisk together eggs, yogurt, and water, then whisk in flour. When blended, stir in cheese, tomato, onion, herbs, salt, and pepper. Pour into the prepared pie dish. Place in oven and bake for 30 minutes or until center is set. Remove from oven and cool on a wire rack for 5 minutes before serving.

◆ CAPONATA FRITTATA ◆

Makes 6 to 8 servings

1 tablespoon olive oil
1/4 cup diced onion
2 cloves garlic, peeled and minced
1 tablespoon minced fresh basil
1 teaspoon minced fresh oregano
1 teaspoon minced fresh parsley
1 1/2 cups diced eggplant
1 cup diced zucchini
1/2 cup diced red bell pepper
1 cup well-drained diced canned plum tomatoes
Salt and pepper to taste
6 large eggs
1/2 cup skim milk
1 cup Yogurt Cheese (page 8)
1/2 cup shredded Monterey Jack cheese

Heat oil in a heavy sauté pan over medium-high heat, then add onion, garlic, and herbs. Sauté for 3 minutes, then add eggplant, zucchini, and bell pepper and sauté for 10 minutes. Add tomatoes, salt, and pepper. Cook for 10 minutes, then remove from heat and allow to cool for 1 hour.

Preheat oven to 350°F.

Spray a 10-inch cast-iron skillet with nonstick vegetable spray.

Beat eggs and milk. Season with salt and pepper and combine with cooled eggplant mixture. Cut yogurt cheese into small pieces and stir in together with Jack cheese. Pour into the prepared skillet. Place in oven and bake for about 40 minutes or until center is set and top is golden. Remove from oven and cool on a wire rack for 5 minutes before cutting.

◆ ASPARAGUS SOUFFLÉ ◆

Makes 6 servings

6 large egg yolks
1/2 cup soft goat cheese
1/2 cup Fromage Blanc (page 9)
Salt to taste
Cayenne pepper to taste
1 1/2 cups diced steamed fresh asparagus
10 large egg whites, stiffly beaten

Preheat oven to 450°F.

Butter a 2-quart soufflé dish. Set aside.

Combine egg yolks, cheeses, salt, and cayenne in a food processor fitted with the metal blade, then pour into a bowl and stir in asparagus. Fold beaten egg whites into asparagus mixture and pour into the prepared soufflé dish. Place in oven and bake for about 20 minutes or until puffed up and golden. Serve immediately.

◆ GARBANZO STEW ◆

Makes 6 servings

1 tablespoon canola oil
2 cups diced onion
2 tablespoons minced garlic
3 cups sliced wild mushrooms
1 1/2 cups diced carrots
1 teaspoon ground cinnamon
1/2 teaspoon ground cumin
2 cups canned plum tomatoes, well-drained
Salt and pepper to taste
4 cups cooked garbanzos (chick-peas), well-drained
1/2 cup pitted Greek olives, well-drained
1/2 cup minced fresh parsley
1/2 cup lemon nonfat yogurt, at room temperature
1 teaspoon fresh lemon juice

Heat oil in a large, heavy saucepan over medium–high heat, then add onions and garlic. Lower heat and sauté for 4 minutes or until onions are just soft. Stir in mushrooms and carrots and sauté for 5 minutes. Add spices and tomatoes and cook for 10 minutes. Season with salt and pepper. Stir in garbanzos, olives, and 1/4 cup parsley and cook for an additional 15 minutes. Stir in yogurt, lemon juice, and remaining parsley. Serve hot with brown rice, if desired.

BREADS AND
◆BREAKFAST TREATS◆

Easy White Bread

Multigrain Bread

Yogurt Chive Cornbread

Yogurt Biscuits

Nan

Yogurt Muffins

Blueberry Muffins

Healthy Muffins

Cinnamon Coffee Cake

Waffles

Buckwheat Pancakes with Sautéed Mushrooms

Oatmeal Pancakes with Fruit Yogurt

◆ EASY WHITE BREAD ◆

Makes 2 loaves

1 cup skim milk
3 tablespoons sugar
Salt to taste
1 cup warm (120°F) water
2 envelopes yeast
1/4 cup plain regular, low-fat, or nonfat yogurt, at room
  temperature
4 1/2 cups all-purpose flour

Place milk, sugar, and salt in a small saucepan over low heat. Cook, stirring constantly, until milk is scalded and sugar and salt are dissolved. Remove from heat and cool to lukewarm.

Place warm water in a large mixing bowl. Stir in yeast until dissolved. Stir in lukewarm milk, then stir in yogurt. Stir in flour a little at a time. The dough will be quite stiff by the time all the flour is incorporated. Use your hands to knead if stirring becomes difficult. When well-blended, cover and let rise in a warm, draft-free spot for about 40 minutes or until doubled in bulk.

Preheat oven to 375°F. Grease 2 9 × 5 × 3-inch loaf pans.

Stir dough down by beating vigorously for about 1 minute. Divide in half and mold each half into the prepared pans. Place in oven and bake for about 40 minutes or until it is cooked in the center and the crust is golden. Remove from oven and from pans. Cool on a wire rack for at least 30 minutes before slicing.

Note: *You may use either vanilla- or lemon-flavored yogurt to give a slight flavor to this bread.*

You can omit the salt and increase the sugar to 1/3 cup for salt-free bread.

When in a hurry, I have often put this bread directly in the oven without a rising period and it has always been light and delicious. I can't guarantee it, but it has worked for me.

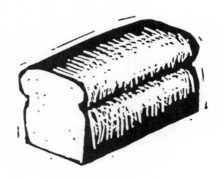

◆ MULTIGRAIN BREAD ◆

Makes 2 loaves

1/2 cup millet
1 cup boiling water
2 cups skim milk
2 tablespoons molasses
1 envelope yeast
1/2 cup plain regular, low-fat, or nonfat yogurt
4 1/2 cups whole-wheat flour
1/2 cup barley flour
1/2 cup rye flour
1/4 cup buckwheat flour
1/2 cup rolled oats
1/2 cup cornmeal
1 tablespoon sea salt

Place millet in a heatproof bowl and pour boiling water over it. Cover and let sit for 30 minutes.

Place milk and molasses in a small saucepan over medium heat, stirring to dissolve molasses. Allow mixture to reach 120°F. If mixture gets hotter, remove from heat and allow to cool down. Stir in yeast. Set aside for 5 minutes, stirring occasionally. Pour into a large mixing bowl. Stir in millet and its soaking water, then stir in yogurt. Combine flours, oats, cornmeal, and salt, then begin stirring into the yeast mixture. The dough will be sticky. When all the flour mixture has been incorporated, turn out onto a clean surface and begin to knead. If the dough is very sticky, add up to 1/2 cup white bread or all-purpose flour. Knead about 10 to 15 minutes or until dough is smooth and elastic.

Lightly grease a large bowl or spray it with nonstick vegetable spray. Put dough in bowl, cover, and let rise in a warm, draft-free spot for about 45 minutes or until doubled in bulk.

Grease and flour two 9 × 5 × 3-inch loaf pans.

Punch dough down and divide in half. Shape into loaves and place in prepared pans. Cover and let rise again in a warm, draft-free spot for about 45 minutes or until doubled in bulk.

Preheat oven to 375°F.

Place loaves in oven and bake for about 50 minutes or until it is cooked in the center and the crust is golden brown. Remove from oven and from pans. Cool on wire racks for at least 30 minutes before cutting.

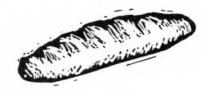

YOGURT CHIVE
◆ CORNBREAD ◆

Makes one 10-inch round loaf

1 1/2 cups all-purpose flour
1 1/2 cups yellow cornmeal
1/4 cup sugar
1 tablespoon baking powder
Salt to taste
1 1/2 cups Imitation Sour Cream (page 9)
3 tablespoons canola oil
2 tablespoons skim milk
1 large egg
1/2 cup chopped fresh chives

Preheat oven to 400°F. Grease a 10-inch cast-iron skillet, or spray it with nonstick vegetable spray. Set aside.

Combine flour, cornmeal, sugar, baking powder, and salt.

Combine imitation sour cream, oil, milk, and egg. Pour into dry ingredients and stir until just moistened. Stir in chives. Pour into prepared skillet. Place in oven, and bake for about 20 minutes or until golden and a cake tester inserted into the center comes out clean. Remove from oven and cool on a wire rack for 5 minutes before cutting.

◆ YOGURT BISCUITS ◆

Makes about 12 biscuits

2 1/2 cups all-purpose flour
1 1/2 cups vanilla nonfat yogurt
1/3 cup sugar
2 tablespoons fine cornmeal
1 tablespoon baking powder
1/2 teaspoon salt
1 tablespoon skim milk

Combine 1 cup flour, 1 cup yogurt, and half the sugar, then cover and set in a warm spot to ferment for 4 hours.

Preheat oven to 425°F.

Lightly grease a 10-inch cast-iron skillet, or spray it with nonstick vegetable spray.

Stir the rest of the flour, yogurt, and sugar and the remaining ingredients into the fermented yogurt until dough just comes together. Add a bit more cornmeal if dough is too sticky, or no more than 1 tablespoon skim milk if dough is too dry. Pat dough into a 1/2-inch thick circle. Using a biscuit cutter or the top of a glass, cut out 12 rounds. Place in the prepared skillet. Put in oven and bake for 12 minutes or until golden. Serve hot.

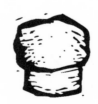

◆ NAN ◆

Makes about 14 breads

1 cup warm (120°F) water
1 envelope yeast
1 tablespoon sugar
1 1/2 cups plain regular, low-fat, or nonfat yogurt, at room temperature
1 teaspoon salt
6 cups bread flour, approximately

Place water in a large mixing bowl and stir in yeast and sugar until well-blended. Set aside for 5 minutes.

Stir in 1 cup yogurt and salt, then begin adding flour, 1 cup at a time, until a firm dough is formed. Knead for about 10 minutes or until dough is smooth and elastic. Place in a lightly greased bowl. Cover and let rise in a warm, draft-free spot for about 45 minutes or until doubled in bulk.

Preheat oven to 500°F. Place a pizza stone, baking tile, or quarry tiles on the lowest rack of the oven. Let heat for 30 minutes.

Punch dough down. Again, knead until it is very smooth, adding flour if necessary to keep dough from sticking. Divide dough into 14 smooth balls. Using your fingertips, flatten each ball into a 6-inch circle. Use a pastry brush to lightly coat the top of each circle with remaining yogurt.

Place circles, a few at a time, onto the hot tiles in oven. Bake for 5 minutes or until puffed and golden. Remove from oven and place on a wire rack to cool.

Note: *You may top this Indian bread with sautéed onions, garlic, or bell peppers, or with grilled, chopped vegetables.*

◆ YOGURT MUFFINS ◆

Makes 12 muffins

1 cup all-purpose flour
1/2 cup extra fine cornmeal
1 teaspoon baking soda
Salt to taste (no more than 1/2 teaspoon)
1 cup vanilla nonfat yogurt
1/4 cup canola oil
1/4 cup pure maple syrup
1/4 cup orange blossom honey
1 teaspoon pure vanilla extract
1 teaspoon freshly grated orange zest
1/2 cup chopped mixed dried fruit
1/4 cup toasted unsalted sunflower seeds

Lightly grease a 12-cup muffin tin, or line with paper liners. Set aside.

Preheat oven to 350°F.

Combine dry ingredients in a medium mixing bowl.

Stir together yogurt, oil, maple syrup, honey, vanilla, and orange zest, then add chopped fruit and sunflower seeds. Stir in dry ingredients to just blend. Spoon into prepared tin. Place in oven and bake for 25 minutes or until golden. Remove from oven and cool on a wire rack.

◆ BLUEBERRY MUFFINS ◆

Makes 12 muffins

1 cup all-purpose flour
1/2 cup cornmeal
1/3 cup sugar
1/2 teaspoon baking powder
1/2 teaspoon baking soda
Salt to taste
3 tablespoons vegetable shortening or soy margarine
1/2 cup vanilla or lemon nonfat yogurt
2 large egg whites
1 teaspoon freshly grated orange zest
1 cup fresh blueberries, washed and dried

Preheat oven to 350°F.

Lightly grease a 12-cup muffin tin, or line with paper liners.

Combine flour, cornmeal, sugar, baking powder, baking soda, and salt, then use your fingers to rub in shortening to make coarse crumbs. Stir in yogurt, egg whites, and orange zest until flour is just smooth. Stir in blueberries. Spoon batter into prepared tin. Place in oven and bake for 20 minutes or until muffins are golden and a cake tester inserted into center of each muffin comes out clean. Remove from oven and tin and cool on a wire rack for 5 minutes before serving.

◆ HEALTHY MUFFINS ◆

Makes 12 muffins

1 cup all-purpose flour
1/2 cup whole-wheat flour
1 cup bran cereal such as All-Bran
1 teaspoon baking powder
1 teaspoon baking soda
2 teaspoons ground cinnamon
1/4 teaspoon ground allspice
1/4 teaspoon ground ginger
1 cup grated carrots
1/2 cup well-drained crushed pineapple
1/2 cup mashed banana
1/2 cup dried cherries
1/4 cup sunflower seeds
2/3 cup vanilla nonfat yogurt
1/2 cup fresh orange juice
1 teaspoon fresh lemon juice
1/4 cup orange blossom honey
2 tablespoons canola oil
1 teaspoon freshly grated orange zest

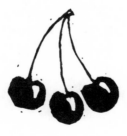

Preheat oven to 350°F.

Line a 12-cup muffin tin with paper liners or spray with nonstick vegetable spray.

Combine flours, bran cereal, baking powder, baking soda, and spices in a mixing bowl.

Combine carrots, pineapple, banana, cherries, sunflower seeds, yogurt, orange juice, lemon juice, honey, oil, and orange zest.

Stir carrot mixture into flour mixture until just moistened. Generously spoon into prepared tin. Place in oven and bake for 20 minutes or until golden and a cake tester inserted into the center of each muffin comes out clean. Remove from oven and tin and cool on a wire rack.

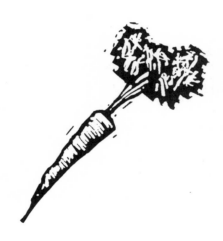

◆ CINNAMON COFFEE CAKE ◆

Makes one 9-inch round cake

3 tablespoons unsalted butter, margarine, or soy
    margarine
3 tablespoons vanilla nonfat yogurt
1 cup sugar
2 large egg whites
2 cups all-purpose flour
1 1/2 teaspoons baking powder
1/2 teaspoon salt or to taste
2 teaspoons ground cinnamon
1 cup skim milk
Cinnamon Topping (recipe follows)

Preheat oven to 350°F.

Grease and flour a 9-inch round cake pan.

Cream together butter and yogurt. Add sugar and beat until well-incorporated. Stir in egg whites. Combine dry ingredients, then stir them into batter, alternating with the milk.

Pour into prepared pan. Sprinkle cinnamon topping on top and cut it into cake with a knife. Place in oven and bake for about 35 minutes or until top is crunchy and a cake tester inserted into the center comes out clean. Remove from oven and cool on a wire rack.

◆ Cinnamon Topping ◆

Makes about 1 1/2 cups

1 cup chopped nuts
1/2 cup light brown sugar
2 tablespoons all-purpose flour
2 tablespoons unsalted butter, margarine, or soy
    margarine
2 teaspoons ground cinnamon

Combine all ingredients, working them into crumbs by rubbing together with your fingertips. Cover and set aside at room temperature until ready to use.

◆ WAFFLES ◆

Makes 8 waffles

2 cups all-purpose flour
5 tablespoons sugar
1 tablespoon baking powder
Salt to taste
2 cups skim milk
1/2 cup vanilla nonfat yogurt
3 tablespoons canola oil
2 large egg whites, stiffly beaten

Combine flour, sugar, baking powder, and salt, then stir in milk, yogurt, and oil. Fold in egg whites. Bake in a hot waffle iron according to manufacturer's instructions. Serve hot with pure maple syrup or fruit toppings.

BUCKWHEAT PANCAKES WITH
◆ SAUTÉED MUSHROOMS ◆

Makes 4 servings

1 teaspoon active dry yeast
1 teaspoon light brown sugar
2 cups warm (120°F) water
1/2 cup all-purpose flour
1 1/2 cups buckwheat flour
Salt to taste
1 tablespoon honey
2 tablespoons plain nonfat yogurt
Sautéed Mushrooms (recipe follows)
1/4 cup chopped fresh chives

Dissolve yeast and sugar in 1/2 cup warm water, then add remaining water. Stir in flours and salt. Blend with a wire whisk to make a thin batter. Cover and allow to rise at room temperature for at least 3 hours or refrigerate overnight. Just before you are ready to cook, whisk in honey and yogurt.

Preheat a nonstick griddle over medium-high heat, then ladle batter onto it to make 3-inch circles. Cook for about 3 minutes or until pancake tops are bubbly and bottoms are light brown. Turn and cook for about 1 minute more or until other side is brown. Remove from heat and keep warm as you continue to make pancakes.

When all pancakes are cooked, place 5 pancakes in a small circle with edges overlapping toward the center of a warm plate. Place about 3/4 cup sautéed mushrooms in the center. Garnish with chopped chives.

◆ Sautéed Mushrooms ◆

Makes approximately 4 cups

6 cups diced fresh mushrooms, preferably a combination
of wild and button mushrooms
1/4 cup minced fresh parsley
1 tablespoon minced onion
1 tablespoon freshly grated orange zest
1/4 cup fresh orange juice
1 tablespoon cognac
Salt and pepper to taste

Place mushrooms, 2 tablespoons parsley, onion, and orange zest and juice in a nonstick skillet over medium-high heat. Cover and allow to come to a boil. Lower heat and continue to just simmer for about 10 minutes or until mushrooms have exuded most of their moisture. Add cognac and continue to cook for 3 minutes. Remove from heat and stir in remaining parsley. Season to taste with salt and pepper. Serve hot.

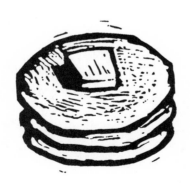

OATMEAL PANCAKES WITH
◆ FRUIT YOGURT ◆

Makes 6 servings

2 cups rolled oats
3/4 cup all-purpose flour
1/3 cup granulated sugar
2 teaspoons baking powder
2 cups buttermilk
1/2 cup plain nonfat yogurt
1 large egg
2 large egg whites, stiffly beaten
2 tablespoons unsalted butter
4 cups sliced peaches, nectarines, apples, or any other
    fruit or berry
2 tablespoons frozen apple juice concentrate, thawed
1 tablespoon light brown sugar
Juice of 1/2 lemon
1 cup fruit-flavored low-fat yogurt

Combine oats, flour, sugar, and baking powder. Stir in buttermilk, plain yogurt, egg, and egg whites, then cover and let rest for 1 hour.

Melt butter in a heavy sauté pan over medium heat, then add fruit. Sauté for 5 minutes. Add apple juice concentrate, brown sugar, and lemon juice. Sauté for 3 more minutes. Remove from heat and keep warm.

Heat a nonstick griddle over medium heat, then drop 1/4 cup batter for each pancake onto the griddle. Cook, turning once, for about 2 minutes per side or until pancakes are cooked through and golden. Keep warm until all pancakes are cooked.

Just before pancakes are ready to serve, stir fruit-flavored yogurt into warm fruit. Serve pancakes with warm fruit on the side.

◆DESSERTS◆

Yogurt Dessert Soup

Yogurt Ice Cream

Easy Homemade Frozen Yogurt

Fruit Mousse

Coeur à la Crème

Yogurt Cheese Cut-out Cookies

Yogurt Cheese Pie

Cheesecake

Almost Good For You Chocolate Cake

Banana Cake

Quick Fruit Cobbler

Poached Fruit with Yogurt Sauce

◆ YOGURT DESSERT SOUP ◆

Makes 6 servings

**4 cups chopped, very ripe cantaloupe, honeydew melon,
    mango, papaya, and peaches
1 cup fresh orange juice
1 tablespoon fresh lime juice
1 cup lemon nonfat yogurt
2 tablespoons julienned fresh mint leaves**

Place fruit and citrus juices in a food processor fitted with
the metal blade and process to form a smooth puree. Pour into a
mixing bowl. Whisk in yogurt until well-combined. Cover and
refrigerate for at least 4 hours or until very cold.

Pour equal portions into six shallow soup bowls and garnish with julienned mint leaves. Serve immediately.

Note: *A small scoop of frozen yogurt in the center of the soup can
be a tasty addition.*

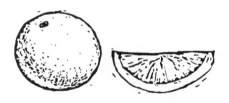

◆ YOGURT ICE CREAM ◆

Makes 1 quart

2 cups plain, vanilla, or lemon nonfat yogurt
2 cups mashed fresh fruit or berries
Scant 1/2 cup extra fine sugar or honey
1 cup heavy cream, whipped

Combine yogurt, fruit, and sugar. Allow to marinate for 10 minutes. Taste and adjust sweetness by adding sugar if necessary. Fold in whipped cream. Pour into an ice-cream freezer and freeze according to manufacturer's instructions. Let stand at room temperature for 20 minutes before serving.

Note: *Omit whipped cream for frozen yogurt. If you have a large 4- to 5-quart ice-cream freezer, double all ingredients.*

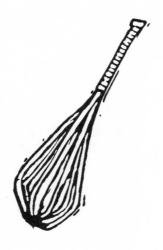

EASY HOMEMADE
◆ FROZEN YOGURT ◆

Makes 6 servings

4 1/2 cups frozen fruit chunks or berries
3/4 cup vanilla or lemon nonfat yogurt
1/2 cup honey or superfine sugar
1 tablespoon fresh orange juice
1 teaspoon fresh lime juice

Combine all ingredients in a food processor fitted with the metal blade. Process until smooth, then pour into a freezer container. Cover and place in the freezer for 1 hour, stirring frequently, or until yogurt mixture is a bit firm and creamy. Serve immediately.

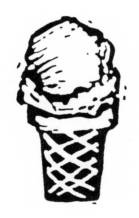

◆ FRUIT MOUSSE ◆

Makes 6 servings

1 cup Yogurt Cheese (page 8)
4 cups pureed cooked fruit such as peaches or apricots
1 3/4 cups fruit juice
2 envelopes unflavored gelatin
1 to 2 tablespoons fruit-flavored liqueur such as Grand
    Marnier or Framboise

Push yogurt cheese through a sieve into pureed fruit. Whisk until well-blended. Set aside.

Bring juice to a boil in a small saucepan over high heat, then whisk in gelatin. Lower heat and whisk until gelatin is dissolved. Pour into fruit mixture. Add liqueur and whisk to combine. Pour into a 1 1/2-quart soufflé dish or individual dessert dishes. Cover and refrigerate for about 4 hours or until well-chilled. Serve, garnished with whipped cream if desired.

Note: *If using peaches or apricots you can use a combination of peach or apricot nectar and orange juice, thinned with water. Always try to use a juice that complements the fruit. Apples and apple cider are terrific.*

◆ COEUR À LA CRÈME ◆

Makes 6 servings

2 cups Yogurt Cheese (page 8)
1 cup sour cream
1/3 cup heavy cream
1/3 cup superfine sugar
1 tablespoon fresh orange juice or pure maple syrup
1 1/2 cups berries, washed and dried
1/3 cup vanilla nonfat yogurt
6 mint sprigs

Beat the cheese, sour and heavy cream, sugar, and orange juice together until very smooth.

Line either a large perforated heart mold or 6 individual perforated heart molds with a double layer of cheesecloth. Place the beaten yogurt mixture into the mold(s). Smooth the top(s) and cover with plastic wrap. Place over a shallow baking dish in a cool spot to drain for at least 8 hours.

When well-drained and firm, uncover, unmold, and peel off cheesecloth. Garnish with fresh berries, yogurt, and mint, or drizzle tops with any flavored syrup.

YOGURT CHEESE
◆ CUT-OUT COOKIES ◆

Makes approximately 4 dozen

1/2 cup Yogurt Cheese (page 8)
1/2 cup unsalted butter, softened
1 cup sugar
1 large egg
1 teaspoon pure vanilla extract
2 to 2 1/2 cups all-purpose flour
3/4 teaspoon baking powder

Cream yogurt cheese and butter. Add sugar and beat until creamy. Add egg and vanilla and beat to blend. Combine 2 cups flour and baking powder. Beat with creamed mixture. Add remaining flour as needed to make a firm dough. Scrape from bowl. Roll into a ball and wrap in plastic wrap. Refrigerate for about 1 hour or until easy to handle.

Preheat oven to 375°F.

When dough is well-chilled, divide in half. On a lightly floured surface, roll out one half at a time to about 1/8 inch thick. Cut out into desired shapes and place, 1 inch apart, on a nonstick cookie sheet. Place in oven and bake for 6 to 8 minutes or until edges are brown. Remove from oven and cool on a wire rack.

Note: *You may sprinkle cookies with cinnamon-sugar or sugar sprinkles before baking, or decorate baked cookies with colored decorator's icing.*

◆ YOGURT CHEESE PIE ◆

Makes one 9-inch pie

3 cups sliced strawberries
1 cup Yogurt Cheese (page 8)
1/2 cup cold water
1 envelope unflavored gelatin
1 tablespoon fresh orange juice
1 teaspoon pure vanilla extract
One 9-inch graham cracker pie shell
1 cup strawberry halves
6 to 8 fresh mint leaves

Blend together strawberries and yogurt cheese in a medium mixing bowl until well-blended. Set aside.

Place water and gelatin in a small saucepan over low heat. Cook, stirring constantly, until gelatin is dissolved. Stir into strawberries. Add orange juice and vanilla and stir to combine. Cover and refrigerate for about 3 hours or until mixture begins to be firm. Scrape into pie shell. Smooth top with a spatula and decorate with strawberry halves and mint leaves. Place in the refrigerator and chill for at least 4 hours before serving.

◆ CHEESECAKE ◆

Makes one 8-inch cake

3/4 cup plain bread crumbs
1/2 teaspoon ground cinnamon
1 cup plus 1 tablespoon sugar
3 cups Yogurt Cheese (page 8)
2 teaspoons pure vanilla extract
3 large eggs
1 cup plain regular, low-fat, or nonfat yogurt
1 to 2 cups fresh fruit such as berries, peeled and sliced
    grapes, kiwi, or peaches

Preheat oven to 375°F.

Combine bread crumbs, cinnamon, and 1 tablespoon sugar. Set aside.

Coat an 8-inch springform pan with nonstick vegetable spray and generously coat pan with bread–crumb mixture.

Cream yogurt cheese, remaining sugar, and vanilla. Add eggs and yogurt and beat until smooth.

Pour into prepared pan and place on the center rack of oven. Bake for 15 minutes, then lower heat to 300°F and bake for another 45 minutes or until the center of the cake has set.

Allow cake to cool in the oven with the door ajar. When cool, remove springform and place cake on a serving plate. Arrange fresh fruit in a decorative pattern on top of cheesecake before serving. Refrigerate until ready to serve.

ALMOST GOOD FOR YOU
◆ CHOCOLATE CAKE ◆

Makes one 9-inch cake

2 cups vanilla nonfat yogurt
1/2 cup soy margarine or any other light vegetable
  spread
1 1/2 cups sugar
1 1/2 cups all-purpose flour
1 cup fine quality cocoa
1 1/2 teaspoons baking soda
1/2 teaspoon baking powder
4 large egg whites
2 tablespoons confectioners' sugar

Spray a 9-inch springform pan with nonstick vegetable spray. Wrap the outside with aluminum foil. Set aside.

Preheat oven to 350°F.

Beat yogurt and margarine with an electric mixer, then add 1 cup sugar, flour, cocoa, baking soda, and baking powder. Beat until mixture is light and fluffy.

Combine egg whites and remaining sugar. Beat until stiff peaks form. Fold into chocolate mixture. Pour into prepared pan. Place filled pan into a larger pan filled with water to come halfway up the sides of the cake pan. Place both pans in oven and bake for about 1 hour or until a cake tester inserted into the center of the cake comes out with only a bit of batter clinging to it. The top of the cake may crack open but this will not affect the taste.

Remove pan from oven and place on a wire rack and cool for 15 minutes. Remove springform and allow cake to cool on the wire rack.

When cool, lightly sift confectioners' sugar over cake. Serve with whipped cream or nonfat frozen yogurt, if desired.

◆ BANANA CAKE ◆

Makes one 9-inch cake

1 cup vanilla nonfat yogurt
3/4 cup mashed very ripe bananas
1 large egg
2 tablespoons canola oil
1 teaspoon freshly grated orange zest
1 1/2 cups all-purpose flour
1/2 cup sugar
2 teaspoons baking powder
1 teaspoon baking soda
1 tablespoon fine quality cocoa
1/2 cup chopped pecans

Preheat oven to 375°F.

Grease and flour a 9-inch square cake pan, or spray it with nonstick vegetable spray.

Place yogurt, bananas, egg, oil, and orange zest in a blender and process until smooth.

Combine flour, sugar, baking powder, baking soda, cocoa, and pecans in a mixing bowl. Pour banana mixture into flour mixture and stir to just combine. Pour into prepared pan. Place in oven and bake for about 20 minutes or until top is light brown and a cake tester inserted into the center comes out clean. Remove from oven and place on a wire rack for 10 minutes. Then turn cake out onto the rack and cool completely before cutting.

◆ QUICK FRUIT COBBLER ◆

Makes 1 cake

4 1/2 to 5 cups peeled, chopped fruit and/or
    well-washed berries (peaches, nectarines, apricots,
    any berry)
1/3 cup firmly packed light brown sugar or to taste
2 tablespoons cornstarch
Juice of 1 lemon
Lemon zest
1 teaspoon ground cinnamon
1/4 teaspoon ground nutmeg
1/2 cup all-purpose flour
1/2 teaspoon baking powder
3 tablespoons vanilla nonfat yogurt
2 tablespoons canola oil
1 tablespoon sugar

Lightly grease an 8-inch round cake pan, or spray it with
nonstick vegetable spray. Combine fruit, brown sugar, cornstarch,
lemon juice and zest, cinnamon, and nutmeg in a medium saucepan
over medium heat. Cook, stirring constantly, for about 7 minutes
or until mixture is just thickened. Scrape into the prepared pan and
set aside.

Preheat oven to 375°F.

Combine flour and baking powder in a small mixing bowl.
Combine 2 tablespoons yogurt and oil, then stir into flour until just
moistened. Shape dough into a ball and pat it out into an 8-inch
circle. Carefully lift circle onto the fruit. Brush top with remaining
yogurt and sprinkle with sugar. Place in oven and bake for about
15 minutes or until top is golden. Remove from oven and cool on
a wire rack for 10 minutes before serving with low-fat or nonfat
frozen yogurt, if desired.

POACHED FRUIT WITH
♦ YOGURT SAUCE ♦

Makes 6 servings

2 cups white wine or water
1 cup sugar or honey
One 2-inch piece orange rind
One 2-inch piece lemon rind
One 3-inch cinnamon stick
6 to 8 whole cloves
4 to 6 cups quartered fresh fruit or 1 pound dried fruit
Yogurt Sauce (recipe follows)

Place wine, sugar, orange and lemon rind, and spices in a heavy saucepan over high heat. Bring to a boil, then lower heat and simmer for about 15 minutes or until a light syrup forms. Add fruit and simmer for about 10 minutes for fresh fruit and about 40 minutes for dried fruit or until fruit is just softened. Remove from heat and allow to cool in syrup. Remove rinds, cinnamon stick, and cloves. Either refrigerate or serve at room temperature with yogurt sauce.

◆ Yogurt Sauce ◆

Makes approximately 2 1/3 cups

1 1/2 cups plain regular, low-fat, or nonfat yogurt
1/2 cup heavy cream
1/3 cup confectioners' sugar
1 tablespoon pure maple syrup
1 tablespoon Grand Marnier

Whisk together all ingredients. Cover and refrigerate until ready to serve.

Note: *You can add 1/2 cup shredded coconut, chopped nuts, and/or raisins to this sauce for extra flavor.*

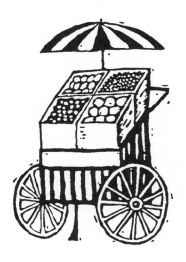

◆A BIT OF EVERYTHING◆

Sauces

Tartar Sauce

Remoulade Sauce

Mustard-dill Sauce

Creole Horseradish Sauce

Parsley-basil Sauce

Spicy Yogurt Sauce

Tahini Sauce

Fresh Carrot Sauce

Dressings

Pesto

Herbed Yogurt Dressing

Guacamole Salad Dressing

Blue Cheese Dressing

500-Island Dressing

Drinks

Fruit Smoothies

Start Your Day Right Breakfast Drink

Lassi

◆ TARTAR SAUCE ◆

Makes approximately 2 cups

1 cup soy or any other mayonnaise
1/2 cup plain regular, low-fat, or nonfat yogurt
1 tablespoon Dijon-style mustard
1/3 cup chopped dill pickles
2 tablespoons chopped capers
1 tablespoon chopped green olives
1 tablespoon minced fresh dill
1 teaspoon minced fresh tarragon
Salt and pepper to taste

Whisk together mayonnaise, yogurt, and mustard, then stir in remaining ingredients. Taste and adjust seasoning. Cover and refrigerate until ready to use.

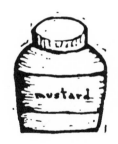

◆ REMOULADE SAUCE ◆

Makes approximately 2 cups

3/4 cup plain nonfat yogurt
3/4 cup soy or any other mayonnaise
2 hard-boiled eggs, peeled and chopped
1 1/2 tablespoons minced fresh parsley
2 cloves garlic, peeled and minced
1 tablespoon bottled horseradish, well-drained
1 tablespoon tarragon-flavored vinegar
1 teaspoon Worcestershire sauce
1/2 teaspoon paprika
1/2 teaspoon dry mustard
Tabasco to taste
Salt to taste

Combine all ingredients until creamy. Taste and adjust seasoning, if necessary. Cover and refrigerate until ready to serve.

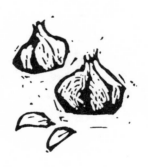

◆ MUSTARD-DILL SAUCE ◆

Makes approximately 1 1/2 cups

1 cup plain regular, low-fat, or nonfat yogurt
3 tablespoons heavy cream
3 tablespoons hot and spicy mustard
3 tablespoons minced fresh dill
1 tablespoon minced shallots
1 teaspoon minced fresh chervil

Whisk all ingredients together. Cover and refrigerate for 30 minutes before using with fish or poultry.

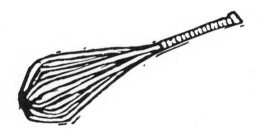

CREOLE HORSERADISH
◆ SAUCE ◆

Makes approximately 1 1/2 cups

1/2 cup plain regular, low-fat, or nonfat yogurt
1/2 cup Imitation Sour Cream (page 9) or any other sour
  cream
1/4 cup prepared horseradish, well-drained
2 tablespoons herb-flavored white wine vinegar
1 1/2 tablespoons Creole mustard
1 teaspoon honey
Tabasco to taste
Salt to taste
1 cup heavy cream, whipped

Whisk together yogurt, sour cream, horseradish, vinegar, mustard, honey, Tabasco, and salt, then cover and refrigerate for 4 hours, or until ready to use. Just before serving, whisk in whipped cream and serve with cold roast meats, poached fish, or grilled or roasted vegetables.

PARSLEY-BASIL
◆ SAUCE ◆

Makes approximately 2 cups

1 cup fresh Italian (flat-leaf) parsley leaves
1/2 cup fresh basil leaves
4 cloves garlic, peeled and minced
1 teaspoon minced green olives
1 cup plain regular, low-fat, or nonfat yogurt

Combine parsley, basil, garlic, and olives in a food processor fitted with the metal blade. Process until smooth. Add yogurt and process until blended. Use as a sauce for salads, meats, poultry, pasta, or rice, or with grilled vegetables.

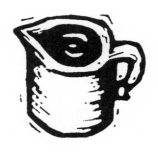

◆ SPICY YOGURT SAUCE ◆

Makes approximately 2 cups

1 cup plain nonfat yogurt
1/4 cup chopped arugula or any other spicy greens
1/4 cup diced red onion
2 cloves garlic, peeled and minced
1 fresh hot green chile, seeded
2 tablespoons chopped cilantro
1 tablespoon chopped fresh mint
Juice of 1 lime
1/4 teaspoon ground cumin
Salt and pepper to taste

Combine yogurt, arugula, and onion in a medium bowl. Place garlic, chile, cilantro, mint, and lime juice in a food processor fitted with the metal blade and process until smooth, then add to yogurt. Stir in cumin, salt, and pepper. Taste and adjust seasoning before serving with fish, poultry, or meats, or on salads, tacos, enchiladas, or burritos.

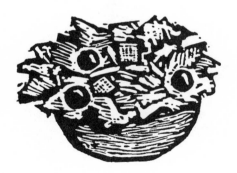

◆ TAHINI SAUCE ◆

Makes approximately 2 cups

1 cup cooked chick-peas (garbanzos), well-drained
1/4 cup plain regular, low-fat, or nonfat yogurt
2 tablespoons tahini (available in Middle Eastern or
   specialty food markets)
4 cloves garlic, peeled and minced
2 tablespoons fresh lemon juice
1/4 teaspoon ground cumin
1/4 teaspoon cayenne pepper or to taste
Salt and pepper to taste

Place chick-peas in a food processor fitted with the metal blade and process until chunky. Add remaining ingredients and process until smooth. If too thick, thin with water or chicken stock. Cover and refrigerate until ready to serve with cold meats or poultry.

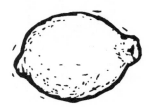

◆ FRESH CARROT SAUCE ◆

Makes approximately 3 cups

4 cups cooked carrots
2 teaspoons fresh lemon juice
1/2 cup plain regular, low-fat, or nonfat yogurt
2 tablespoons minced cilantro
Tabasco to taste
Salt to taste

Puree carrots with lemon juice in a food processor fitted with the metal blade. When smooth, scrape into a small bowl. Whisk in remaining ingredients, then cover and refrigerate for 1 hour before serving with cold meats, poultry, or fish.

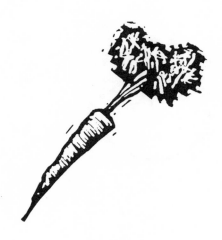

◆ PESTO ◆

Makes approximately 1 1/2 cups

2 cups fresh basil leaves
1/4 cup extra virgin olive oil
2 tablespoons toasted pine nuts
2 cloves garlic, peeled and minced
1/4 cup grated Parmesan cheese
1/2 cup plain regular, low-fat, or nonfat yogurt
Salt to taste

Combine basil, olive oil, nuts, and garlic in a food processor fitted with the metal blade. When blended, add Parmesan and yogurt and process until smooth. Taste and adjust seasoning with salt, if necessary. Serve at room temperature with pasta, on salads, or with fish or poultry.

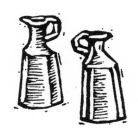

◆ HERBED YOGURT DRESSING ◆

Makes approximately 2 1/2 cups

1 cup plain nonfat yogurt
1 cup lightly packed arugula or watercress
2 tablespoons minced fresh basil
2 tablespoons minced fresh parsley
2 tablespoons minced fresh dill
2 tablespoons minced fresh celery leaves
2 tablespoons minced scallion
1 tablespoon minced fresh mint
1 tablespoon pure maple syrup
1 teaspoon fresh lime juice
Salt and pepper to taste

Combine all ingredients in a food processor fitted with the metal blade and process until smooth. Cover and refrigerate until ready to use. Serve chilled on salads, sandwiches, or vegetables.

GUACAMOLE SALAD
◆ DRESSING ◆

Makes approximately 1 1/2 cups

1 very ripe avocado, peeled and seeded
1/2 cup plain nonfat yogurt
Juice of 1 lime
1/2 fresh hot green chile or to taste
1 clove garlic, peeled and minced
2 tablespoons chopped cilantro
2 tablespoons chopped red onion

Combine avocado, yogurt, lime juice, chile, and garlic in a food processor fitted with the metal blade. When smooth, pour into a small bowl. Stir in cilantro and onion. Cover and refrigerate until ready to serve.

◆ BLUE CHEESE DRESSING ◆

Makes approximately 1 3/4 cups

1 cup plain nonfat yogurt
1/2 cup crumbled blue cheese
3 tablespoons milk
2 tablespoons raspberry vinegar
1 clove garlic, peeled and minced
1 teaspoon minced fresh thyme
1 teaspoon pure maple syrup

Combine all ingredients until well-blended and chunky. Cover and refrigerate until ready to serve.

◆ 500-ISLAND DRESSING ◆

Makes approximately 3 cups

1 cup plain regular, low-fat, or nonfat yogurt
2 ripe tomatoes, peeled, seeded, chopped, and well
    drained
3 tablespoons diced red bell pepper
3 tablespoons chopped fresh chives
2 tablespoons chopped pickles of choice
1 tablespoon minced cilantro
1 tablespoon pure maple syrup
Salt and pepper to taste

Combine all ingredients, then cover and refrigerate until
ready to serve.

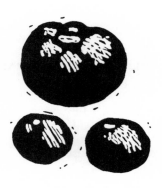

◆ FRUIT SMOOTHIES ◆

Makes 2 servings

1 cup plain, vanilla, or lemon nonfat yogurt
2 cups fruit, frozen
1/2 cup fresh orange juice

Place yogurt in the freezer for 1 hour, then put in a blender with remaining ingredients and process until thick and smooth. Serve immediately.

Note: *Frozen strawberries or bananas, separately or in combination, make particularly refreshing smoothies.*

START YOUR DAY RIGHT
◆ BREAKFAST DRINK ◆

Makes 2 servings

1 1/2 cups plain, vanilla, or lemon yogurt
1 peeled banana, frozen
Juice of 2 oranges
1 tablespoon fresh lemon juice
2 tablespoons silken tofu
1 tablespoon honey
1 tablespoon wheat germ

Combine all ingredients in a blender, then pour into tall glasses and serve immediately.

◆ LASSI ◆

Makes 4 to 6 servings

2 cups plain or lemon nonfat yogurt
6 ice cubes
1 1/2 cups ice water
1 tablespoon fresh lemon juice
1 tablespoon fresh orange juice
3 tablespoons superfine sugar or honey

Process yogurt, ice cubes, ice water, and juices in a blender for 30 seconds. Add sugar and process for about 1 minute or until smooth. Serve over ice and garnish with a mint sprig, if desired.

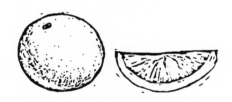

◆ INDEX ◆